New Beginnings

The Triumphs of 120 Cancer Survivors

Photographs by Bill Aron
Text edited by Bill Aron, Bill Kavanagh and Susan Carrier

Foreword by Jane E. Brody

Prefaces by Peter Yarrow, U.S. Representative Henry Waxman
and Rabbi David J. Wolpe

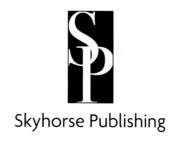

Skyhorse Publishing

Skyhorse Publishing books may be purchased in bulk at special discounts for sales promotion, corporate gifts, fund-raising, or educational purposes. Special editions can also be created to specifications. For details, contact the Special Sales Department, Skyhorse Publishing, 307 West 36th Street, 11th Floor, New York, NY 10018 or info@skyhorsepublishing.com.

Skyhorse® and Skyhorse Publishing® are registered trademarks of Skyhorse Publishing, Inc.®, a Delaware corporation.

Visit our website at www.skyhorsepublishing.com.

10 9 8 7 6 5 4 3 2 1

Library of Congress Cataloging-in-Publication Data is available on file.

Cover design by Jane Sheppard
Cover Photograph by Bill Aron

Print ISBN: 978-1-63220-664-0
Ebook ISBN: 978-1-63220-888-0

Printed in China

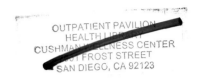
To the memory of our parents:

Eva and Samuel Aron
and
Sylvia and Moshe Ettenberg

Contents

Foreword

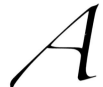As is often said of old age, having—and living after—cancer is not for sissies. But surprising though it may seem, and as Bill Aron's book aptly demonstrates, many—perhaps most—people who survive the experience end up tougher, braver, more resilient and more compassionate than they were going in.

A cancer diagnosis is unquestionably a comeuppance. Few expect it and for most it is a life-changing experience that derails any preexisting intimations of immortality. Suddenly there is, for many, a need to make each day count, to not postpone important goals, and often to do things that might leave a life-enhancing lasting legacy.

It doesn't necessarily have to be your own cancer for such a dramatic redirection of philosophy and action to occur. I was sixteen and about to graduate from high school when my mother succumbed at age forty-nine to ovarian cancer. I vowed then to do what I could to avenge her untimely death by helping others lead healthy, productive, and hopefully longer and fulfilling lives. And I pursued that goal like a horse with blinders for the rest of my life.

By the time I got cancer sixteen years ago at age fifty-seven, I wasn't even scared. I considered it a speed bump, not a roadblock. I didn't ask "Why me?" Why not me? Just because I eat a wholesome diet and exercise every day and have never smoked or overindulged in alcohol does not render me immune to cancer. And even if you think something avoidable that you did had resulted in your cancer, nothing good can come from recriminations about the past. Rather than beating up on yourself, focus on what good can lie ahead.

In preparing a talk I gave to cancer survivors and their families, I looked up some inspiring quotes from others who have been through a cancer experience. I found very helpful statements like these:

"Life isn't about waiting for the storm to pass, it's about learning to dance in the rain."

"We don't know how strong we are until being strong is the only choice we have."

When I received a diagnosis of breast cancer, my first thought was *It's not about the breast*. Rather, it's about health in its totality. It's about life and how you approach it.

I had already left behind a body of work that would remain meaningful to millions of others for decades to come. And I vowed to do what I could to keep that legacy growing for as long as possible. I also continued to pursue the lesson I learned from my mother's early death—don't put off for some indefinite future what you want to do and can do today.

Knowing full well that whatever I had earned could not follow me into the Great Beyond, I chose to help others, both at home and abroad, pursue the kind of education I had been privileged to obtain. I articulated explicit values and put my assets to work to support them for my young relatives and for countless young people I don't know and probably never will. I don't believe in squandering money on fancy cars, boats, clothes and jewelry when so many people in this country and in the world go to bed each night hungry and without a secure roof over their heads, when so many children in the world don't have a book to read or the ability to read one if they did.

I'm not suggesting everyone adopt my particular set of values or approach to life. But I am saying that whether it's cancer or some other life-threatening condition you or a loved one might have, it behooves you to take stock before it's too late and decide, as I did at sixteen, to live each day as if it could be your last, all the while with an eye on the future in case it isn't.

Whether you are destined to live weeks, months, years or decades after a cancer diagnosis, you will have achieved nothing worthwhile for yourself or others unless it changes your life for the better. I know scores of people who are cancer survivors. Some are living with cancer. Some, at the moment at least, are cancer-free. Others seem to have beaten the disease many years ago. The one characteristic that unites them all is a determination to make their remaining time on earth meaningful to themselves, their loved ones and many others they'll never meet.

Perhaps the most inspiring cancer patient I know is Wendy Schessel Harpham. Like the many survivors in this book, Wendy focuses on hope, not hope for a cure but hope for long, productive survival. Wendy is a physician living in Dallas. She was in her thirties, the mother of three young children and loving her medical practice when in 1990 she learned she had non-Hodgkin's lymphoma. Wendy has had cancer now for twenty-five years. She's currently in a long remission but has endured many rounds of treatment, some of them highly experimental, for periodic recurrences—eight of them to date.

Wendy's goal is to get the best treatment available, live as long as she can, and, most important, live as fully as she can every single day. When Wendy's illness forced her to give up her beloved medical practice, she turned to writing terrific books to help others through the ordeal of cancer. She also appears on national television, speaks to both lay and professional audiences about cancer survival, writes a blog for patients and their families and a column for oncologists to help them deal more sensitively with their patients.

Wendy has written: "Cancer made it impossible for me to practice medicine, then led me to discover a different but equal passion and a way to reach more people than I ever could in my office."

In other words, Wendy has turned a sow's ear into a silk purse. Every cancer survivor has the potential to follow her example.

Conquering cancer is really not about cure. It's about living—living well for as long and as fully as one can. Wendy, who has had more experience and expertise at surviving cancer than most, calls it a journey. Journeys can be challenging, long, and difficult. But they can also be life-enhancing. How each person weathers the journey is a matter of choice. You can choose to rant and rail at the misfortune that found you, or you can make the most of however much time you have left and, in the end, be able to write your own epitaph—an epitaph that would make others proud to have known you or wishing they had.

As Wendy put it, cancer is not a battle and it's not a war. Wars, whatever their outcome, are horrific experiences that leave behind unimaginable devastation. A journey, on the other hand, can be meaningful and often joyful in and of itself.

This book can help you make it so.

Jane E. Brody
Personal Health columnist
The New York Times
New York, NY

Preface

ancer is a major public health problem in the United States. Diagnoses directly affect one in four Americans. The number of new diagnoses in 2014 is expected to be 1,665,540, up from 1,437,180 in 2008. Moreover, medical expenses are one of the leading causes of bankruptcy in the country.

This is a problem that runs deeply through nearly every family in America.

The bright spot is that the cancer death rate for both men and women combined has declined 20 percent from 1991 to 2010. More than 1.3 million cancer deaths have been averted in that time frame as a result of this decline.

New Beginnings consists of interviews and emotionally expressive portraits of 120 cancer survivors, ages two through ninety-nine. We hear in their own words the struggles they've experienced as we come to understand how their lives have been changed in a positive way.

Their words move us as we share their triumphs; the photographs become inspiring visual interpretations of their feelings. Together, the words and photographs set a context for understanding how people persevere in the face of serious illness. Dr. Thomas R. Frieden, director of the Centers for Disease Control, reflects, "Having cancer may be the first stage, really, in the rest of your life."

Bill Aron's *New Beginnings* sensitively portrays that first stage, thus making a significant contribution to the growing field of survivorship.

US Representative Henry Waxman
Washington, DC

Preface

By Peter Yarrow

*T*his is a book for all of us: cancer patients, survivors and, equally so, for those who might never face that challenge. As only art can, Bill Aron's book informs the part of us that is willing to believe, to care, to do whatever is necessary to turn a terminal threat into a celebration of victory. We emerge from this book's journey knowing that a miracle is within the reach of all of us, not only in terms of the survival and triumph over cancer, but in terms of how this experience can become a source of inspiration and a great teacher.

Bill Aron rallies people's hearts, not to only to commit, with all their might, to taking on the daunting challenge of defeating cancer, but he also rallies those on the outside, who are the families and extended families of these brave cancer warriors of this book. They survive cancer to become blessed angels in our midst.

We learn that the most daunting challenges teach us that the essence of life is not at all what we once supposed. A new awareness emerges that intellectually, cannot be fully understood. It can, however, be experienced in the faces of the subjects of this book along with their unvarnished words; together they convey the great gift of Bill Aron's book.

Peter Yarrow, 2014
New York City

By Rabbi David J. Wolpe

*B*ill Aron *sees*. Where most of us walk through the day capturing glimpses and being periodically arrested by an interesting face or an unusual sight, rare is the individual for whom the surface reveals depths. I am grateful to have my picture in this book not only because it means I survived, but because Bill has created a tribute, a glorious celebration of overcoming.

What you hold is both an exploration and an inspiration. Here are the stories of people who found the way through; they were fortunate in medicine to be sure, but also in spirit. Each page teaches a new lesson in adjusting to and embracing what life presents. Reading through each exploration and seeing the photo is the inspiration: you see, through Bill's artistic eye, how each life has been shaped by the crucible of cancer.

I invite you to a wonderful pageant. In this beautiful book you get to meet 120 lucky people who have been granted the chance to begin again.

Rabbi David J. Wolpe
Los Angeles, CA

Acknowledgments

Contrary to what most people think, photography is not a solitary experience.

Many people helped me bring this project to fruition. Most important are the participants whose stories and images fill these pages. I was welcomed not only into their homes, but also into their hearts. They gave me a gift of openness and trust, which made possible 120 truly memorable encounters. It was the essence of these encounters, a deep sense of connection that I felt and that I tried to put into the images. The extent to which my photographs succeed is due to their spirit.

When I first conceptualized this project in 2006, I was not sure how or where I might find survivors who were willing to open up to me. The Wellness Community, now called the Cancer Support Community, provided me with a few names with which to try out my ideas. I also scoured the social media sites on the Internet. I wanted to skew the project toward younger survivors and found Planet Cancer, a social media site for people under forty who have been diagnosed with cancer. I also found a sympathetic friend in Dr. Leonard Sender, Medical Director of the Hyundai Cancer Institute at the Children's Hospital of Orange County, who introduced me to wonderful families of young children and teenagers. In a relatively short time, other survivors who heard about the project began contacting me, saying they wanted their experience to help others. Still others, I sought out because of their unique contributions to the cancer survivor community. I still have a folder full of names, and could have continued this work indefinitely. It was time however, to call cloture.

Throughout the past eight years, many foundations and friends, through applications, letter writing and crowd sourcing, generously donated financially to this project, thereby lending much needed material and moral support. I am extremely grateful. They are:

Veronica Abney

Melinda Smith Altshuler

Angell Foundation

Anonymous

Gay Block

Nadine and Steve Breuer

Adele Lander Burke and Rick Burke

Sunny Caine

Fran Chalin

Nora and Andy Chapkis

Mat and Donna Chazinov

Toni and Bruce Corwin

Rhea Coskey

Gary Culpepper

Patricia Czoschke

Vivian and Philip Deutsch

Drs. Gail and Sheldon Dorph

Ben B. and Joyce Eisenberg Foundation

Jackie and David Ellenson

In Memory of Sylvia Ettenberg

Janet and Jake Farber

Rabbi Nina Bieber Feinstein and Rabbi Ed Feinstein

Leora Fishman

Michael Forman

Rabbi Karen Fox and Mickey Rosen

Charles J. Frankel, MD

Georgia and Gary Freedman-Harvey

Jean & Dr. Jerry Friedman

Christina and Christian Fuhrer

Cindy and Neil Garroway

Haim Geffen

Beverly and Herbert Gelfand

Rabbi Laura Geller and Richard Siegel

Sharon Gillerman and Mark Quigley

Sharon and Herbert Glaser
Paul Cary Goldberg
Roslyn and Abner Goldstine
Paul Goldenberg
Laurie Goodman and Don Spetner
Cantor Judy and Michael Greenfeld
Adele and Bert Greenspun
Marlene and Marshall Grossman
Grace and Ira Grossman
Dorien Grunbaum
Jackie Gutwirth and Misha Avramoff
Janet R. Halbert
Naomi and Mordechai Hanochi
Kathryn Hellerstein and David Stern
Miriam Prum Hess and and Mark Hess
The Hitter Family Foundation
Ruth and Gershon Hundert
Elisa Hunziker
Shirley and Aubrey Hyman
Jonathan Jacoby
Judith Kandel
Diane and John Katz
Madelyn Katz
Corie and Michael Koss
Rabbi Susan Laemmle and John Antignas
Alice and Nahum Lainer
Ellie and Mark Lainer
Peachy and Mark Levy
Lewis Family Foundation
Kayla and Joel Mandelbaum
Amy Mates and Billy Mencow
Anne Tavan and Rabbi Rim Meirowitz
Ruth and Dan Merritt
Alan Metnick
Shirley and Alan Molod
Katherine Moore
Todd Morgan
Rocky and Lon Morton
Esther Netter
Elisa Newman, MD
Perry Oretzky
Ilene and Jeff Nathan, In memory of Jan Lasky Platt

Janet and David Polak
Helen Randall and Frank Ponder
Riv-Ellen Prell and Steven Foldes
Sylvia Price
Adele and Herbert Reznikoff
Judith Rivin
Zoe Robinson
The Rogers Foundation
J. P. Roos
Marilyn Rosen
Gayle Garner Roski
Alissa and Warren Roston
Brad Rumble
Wendy and Ken Ruby
Laurence Salzmann
David Sampliner
Ellen and Richard Sandler
Michal Scharlin
Joan Scherman
Fred Schor
Sandy and Marvin Schotland
Lisa and Mark Schwartz
Kathryn Scruggs
Freda Foh Shen
Doni Silver Simons
Terri and Michael Smooke
Jay and Deanie Stein Foundation
Gretchen and Jay Stein
Susan and Joel Stern
Ann Stephens
Judith and Art Tischler
Justine Trueger
Gila and Dove Vogel
Mickey and Judge Joseph Wapner
Michael Waterman
Edna and Mickey Weiss Family Foundation
Harriet Zeitlin
Marcie and Howard Zelikow
Tali and Benny Zelkowicz
Elana and Scott Zimmerman
Marshall S. Zolla

There are a few people without whom this project would be years away from completion. I am forever in their debt for their belief in and support of this idea from the first interviews to the last. Gretchen and Jay Stein, Nancy Berman and Alan Bloch, I cannot thank you enough.

No list of thanks would be complete without the mention of Michael States, Rabbi Rim Meirowitz, and Professor William Cutter, whose wisdom guided me both personally and professionally, urging me on toward the next step, while gently talking me through the many problems along the way. Thanks are also due to Eliot Ivanhoe, whose needles kept me going, and to Howard Mendelson, MD, who advised me on all the medical terminology. And along the way, my oncologists, Mark Scholz, MD, and Richard Lam, MD, looked after my health.

I am particularly indebted to Freda Foh Shen who introduced me to photography. Without her, I would never have picked up a camera.

Sue and Bernie Pucker of the Pucker Gallery in Boston, from the earliest days of our relationship, have always believed in and encouraged my work. That has meant a lot to me.

Bill Kavanagh and Susan Carrier took the spoken words from the interviews and turned them into much better prose. It has been a pleasure working with you. Also, Lilia Arbona, friend and extraordinary designer, helped me throughout the project to see the text and images as a book.

I wish also to thank Bonny Fetterman who shepherded my manuscript through the myriad of conversations with publishers. Her patience with them, and with me, was infinite.

Over the course of this project I had two amazing photography assistants who anticipated all of my photographic needs. Thank you Alexis Stein and Pablo Serrano. I also had essential guidance from Richard Maier, my Photoshop and "all things Mac" guru.

Not least of all, I wish to thank Jane Sheppard and the design team, and my editors, Alexandra Hess and Joseph Sverchek at Skyhorse Publishers. I know I was perhaps overly obsessive of the details, but you guided the book through its creation with grace. I am extremely proud of our final product.

I had many photography teachers, both in person and by example. I feel special gratitude to the magnificent portraiture and brilliant compositions of Arnold Newman, Brian Lanker and my teacher, Philippe Halsman, as well as to the glorious and uninhibited spirit of Robert Frank and the versatility of Joel Meyerowitz.

Most of all, I thank and dedicate this book to my wife and my friend, Isa Aron, as well as to my two sons, Hillel and Jesse, for their encouragement, support and love. I could not have done any of this without all of you to come home to.

INTRODUCTION

"Y ou have cancer" are three terrifying words, but our culture does little to ease the fear. *New Beginnings: The Triumph of 120 Cancer Survivors* follows 120 survivors who discovered that those words were the start of a new beginning, not an end to their lives. Their stories inspire and provide hope for anyone diagnosed with cancer, their families and their friends.

New Beginnings explores the question of what happens during the *"silent phase" after treatment ends.* That's when the frenetic flurry of treatment and doctors' appointments is replaced with a huge anomic silence. Even families and friends tend to see the conclusion of treatment as an "end." At this point, survivors are left to their own resources as they attempt to move forward. But, as Dr. Thomas R. Frieden, director of the Centers for Disease Control, reflects, "Having cancer may be the first stage, really, in the rest of your life."

Cancer forces people to put their lives on hold. It can cause physical and emotional pain, and result in lasting problems. It may even end in death. But many people gain a new perspective on life. It is as if their senses become more finely tuned by facing their own mortality. The fragility as well as the strength that survivors feel is the story I hope to convey through this book.

I wish that this book had existed when I was diagnosed with prostate cancer in 1993 when I was fifty-two years old. There was no Internet then, so I went to a medical library and came away terrified. When the cancer returned after surgery and fourteen months of remission, I thought that the rest of my life would be hell. The subsequent chemotherapy and radiation may have been difficult, but they were nothing compared to how I felt emotionally.

Adjusting to my diagnosis of cancer took some time and the help of a gifted therapist. I became aware of what really mattered. I focused on what I loved about my work, and minimized what I disliked. I strove to make my family and friends a bigger part of my life. I became a better husband, father and friend. Cancer became, as many survivors concur, the worst and best gift I ever received—the catalyst for accepting my limitations, my mortality, and my strengths. I learned that fear, pain and depression do not have to be lasting events, but can be viewed as passages to somewhere and something better. I had the opportunity for a new beginning. The creation of this book initiated that process.

I began my career as a photographer during the heyday of black and white street photography. I was fascinated by how people moved and interacted with each other. In order to give expression to that idea, I had to overcome all hesitancy about confronting people with my camera. Once I began to enlist the cooperation of subjects, I fell in love with portraiture, with saying something substantive about the person in front of my lens. The portraits in *New Beginnings* are a reflection of my desire to give subjects the freedom to interact with me through gesture, expression and conversation.

New Beginnings is a collection of narratives and "energetic" photographic portraits of men, women, and families of children. They vary in age, ethnicity and diagnosis, but they all share the ability to turn a diagnosis of cancer into a positive force in their lives. This is a project by and for cancer survivors: their words, my photographs in collaboration with their sensibilities.

The survivors portrayed in this book are vibrant, fully alive in spirit, mind, and body, in spite of the obstacles they have encountered. They may be ordinary people, but their triumph over their struggles is heroic. In the words of Megan, age eighteen:

When they told me the news, it was the worst day of my life. Everything after that got easier. It made me who I am, and I like the person I am today.

This is their book.

Bill Aron

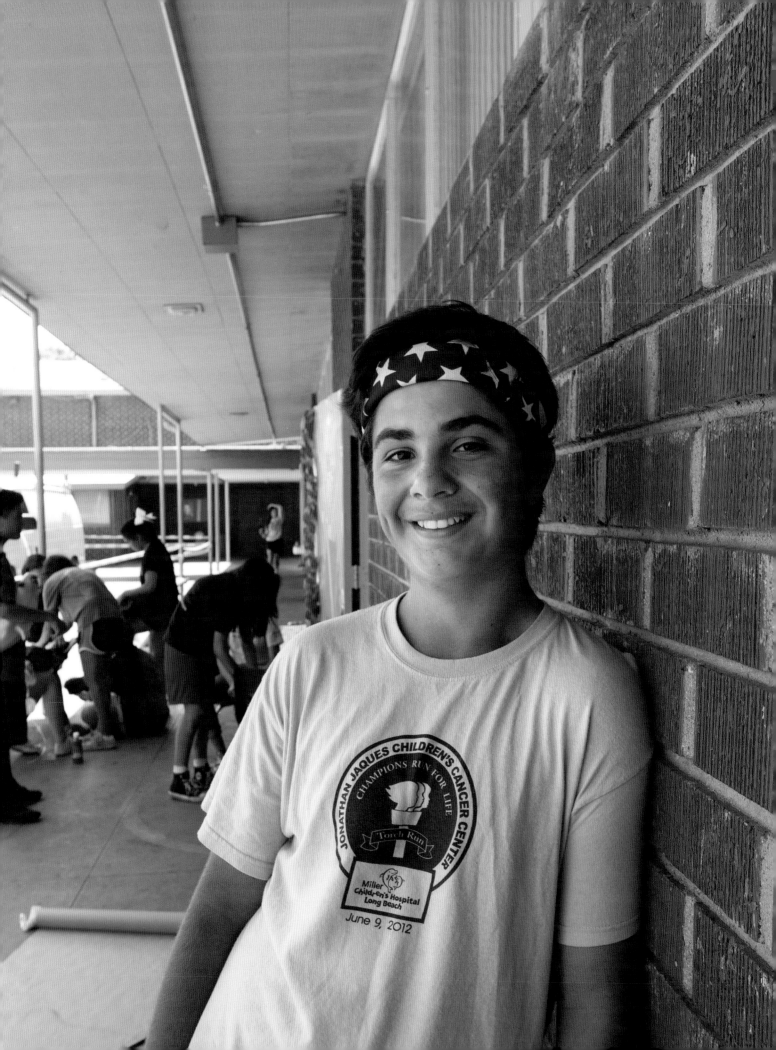

Aaron Rutz | Age at diagnosis, 9
Chronic myelogenous leukemia, 2007

AARON: September 21, 2007, was a day that changed my life forever. My parents took me into their bedroom to tell me the news. My first reaction was, "You're kidding, right?" I didn't know what it was, but I had seen kids on TV with cancer. I knew it was serious.

It became hard to do even the simplest things. I missed two years of school, sports, and social activities. Hospital stays and constant worry about my health replaced the fun that most nine year olds have. The Lakers point guard Jordan Farmar came to see me one day in the hospital, but I couldn't even wake up to talk to him. That shows how sick I was at the time.

MARY, AARON'S MOTHER: We went from a happy, normal family to our worst nightmare realized. It was the worst day of my entire life. Aaron had a very rare type of leukemia for children—one in a million. His brother Adam was a match for his bone marrow, so he had the transplant just a few months later. When he started losing his hair, he cut it into a Mohawk. His father, his brothers, and several of his friends all had their heads shaved in solidarity.

> If you ever wonder "Where are all the good people in the world?" they are in pediatric oncology.

MICHAEL, AARON'S FATHER: I now know what it is like to beg God for the life of a child. His brother Adam was heroic. He called and emailed so many people, including our church, and asked for prayers. He told the pastor, "I don't know what it costs to have a special Mass said, but I'll pay for it to make my brother well."

MARY: When normality returned, we were so happy. If I see my kids fighting, I feel the joy of them being normal, and I let them fight. We pray together every night as a family. We pray for all the kids in the hospital. The silver lining is that we found all the goodness in people who helped us at every stage. If you ever wonder "Where are all the good people in the world?" they are in pediatric oncology.

In 2013 Aaron completed his freshman year in high school, maintaining a 4.0 GPA. He also accomplished his dream of making the baseball team and was voted "Player of the Year" by his teammates. He values every single opportunity he has to step out on the field.

Aaron now has hopes to go to med school to become a pediatric hematologist-oncologist. He says he has learned to take it one day at a time.

MARY: I now know that heaven is when you get your every hope and dream, and it turns out better than you could have ever imagined.

1

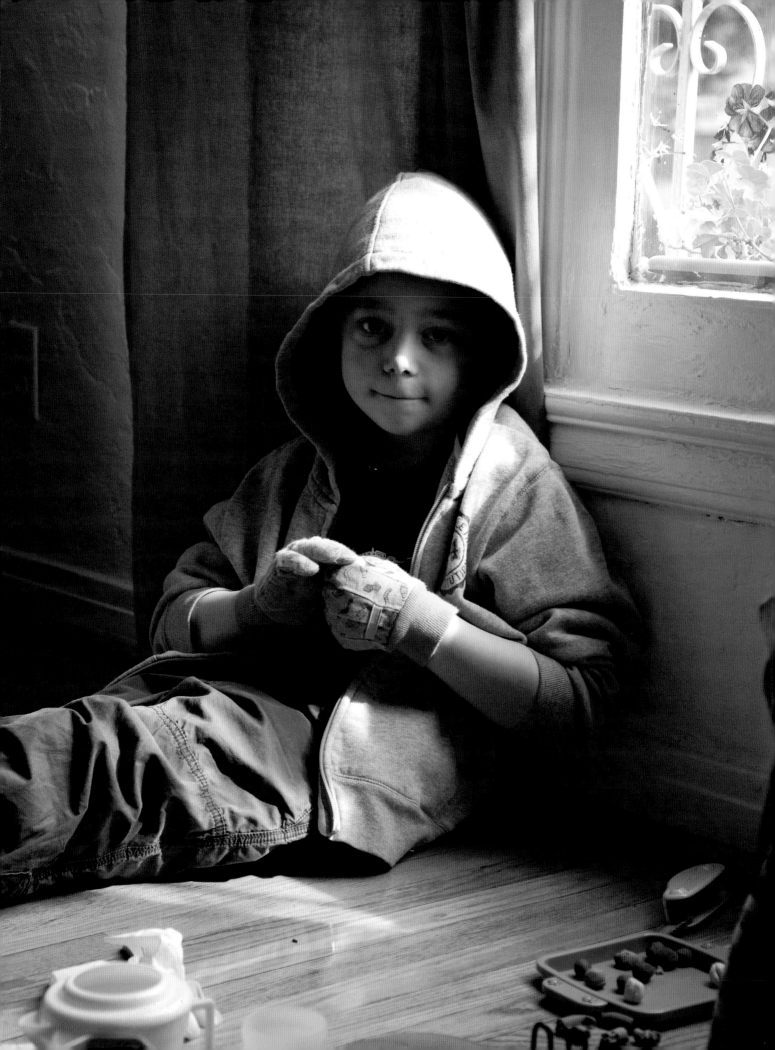

Adam Pomerantz

Age at diagnosis, 6
Leukemia, 2008

SHAROE, ADAM'S FATHER: In the beginning you ask, "Why us?" And then eventually you start to thank God for all the things you do have. We decided to take the good things from this experience and make our lives better. It even transferred to my business—looking for all the good things. Everywhere I go now, I look at all that we have, not what's missing.

> Everywhere I go now, I look at all that we have, not what's missing.

SHARON, ADAM'S MOTHER: After Adam was diagnosed, we were going to move back to Israel because we had only lived in this country for seven months. And then we got amazing support. We had never known a community like this before. We are so lucky that we found all of these amazing people.

Thanks to Adam's cancer I find myself choosing my battles differently. The experience "rounded" me and helped me go with the flow more than I was ever able to do before. We now *know* what's really important and what's not. Even Adam says he feels grateful, and he talks about all the good things that came about from his having had leukemia.

> We now know what's really important and what's not.

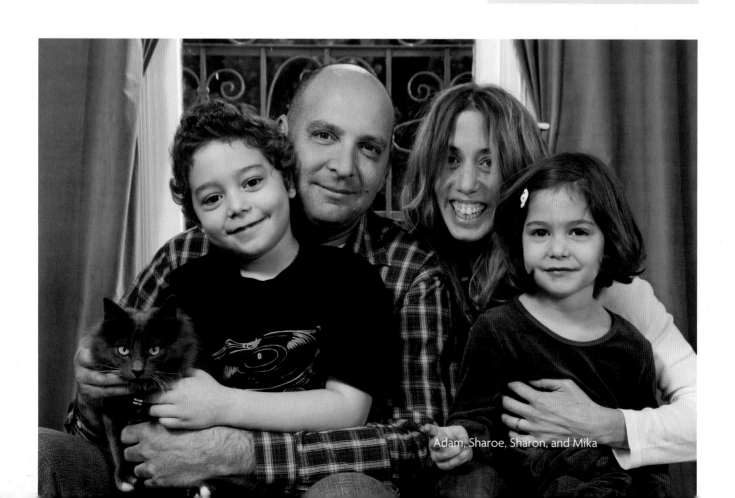

Adam, Sharoe, Sharon, and Mika

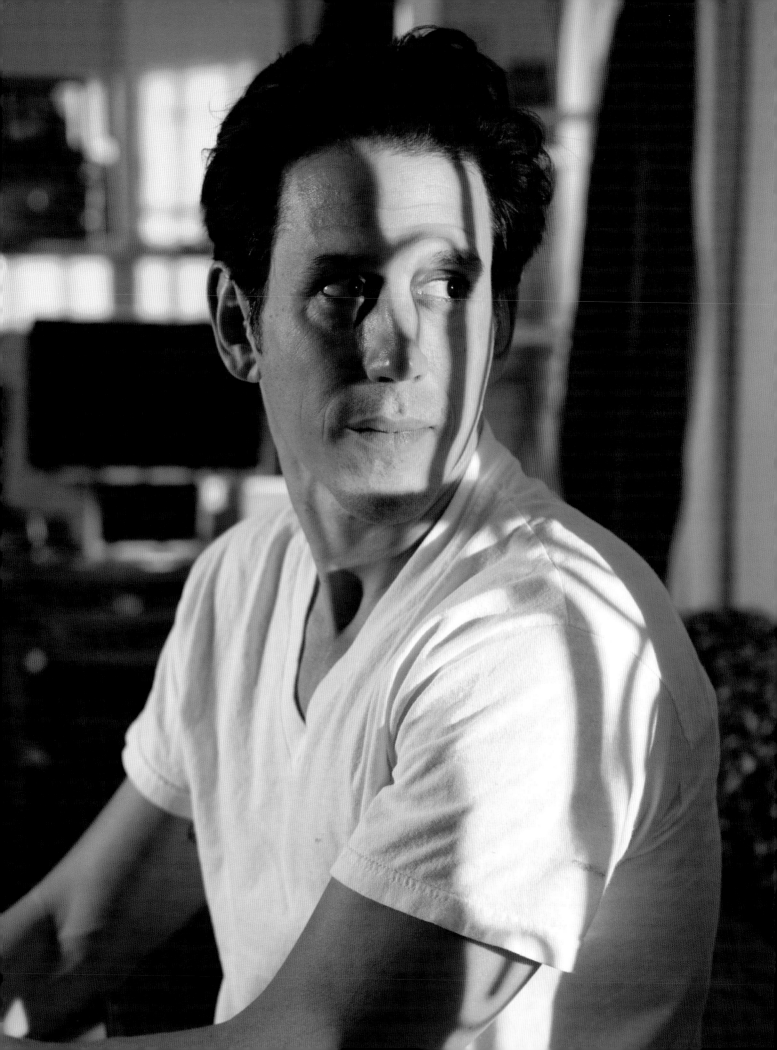

Adam Tomei

Actor, Writer, Producer
Age at diagnosis, 36
Fibromyxoid sarcoma, 2002

So many factors cause cancer, but they have no idea of the source of mine. It wasn't genetic or environmental, and it's a very rare form. They did know that it was life threatening. Those are heavy words.

On Valentine's Day, my doctor's office called and said, "You have a large lump on your leg, and it could very well be cancer." That was the same day that I got my divorce papers. So whenever anyone tells me they've had a bad Valentine's Day, I say, "Really? Let me tell you about one that I had."

Everything was going to be new and different. And then in the end, I realized that I liked my life.

I knew that my parents would be freaked out. I've given them a lot of trouble in my lifetime, and I didn't want this to be another thing for them to worry about. Losing a child is the worst thing that can happen to parents. I didn't want my parents and sister, who is my best friend, to have to deal with my not being alive.

I had the surgery, then chemo and radiation. I also went to an acupuncturist, a kabbalist, a psychic, and an Eastern medicine specialist. I just wanted to throw the kitchen sink at it. I figured it couldn't hurt.

Friends of mine from college sent a letter to everyone I know. Their goal was to get 180 pages of good wishes for my 180 days of chemo. I got responses from many people who I hadn't heard from in many years. Several of them took me to my chemo treatments, which became like a talk show. We would laugh so much, the hospital often had to tell us to keep it down.

A big part of my recovery came from lessons I learned in a twelve-step program. When I was at my lowest, the teachings helped me focus on one day at a time. Instead of self-pity I just tell myself, *Well, you're not dead.*

Good Morning, This is God! I will be handling all your problems today. I will NOT need your help - so, have a good day.

I went through crazy, grandiose ideas that I was going to change my life. I remember thinking that if they cut off my leg, I could become the first one-legged president. Everything was going to be new and different. And then in the end, I realized that I liked my life.

The one real change that I made was a new sense of gratitude, an appreciation for life. Just life. Just being alive. I never had that before. Now I feel it all the time.

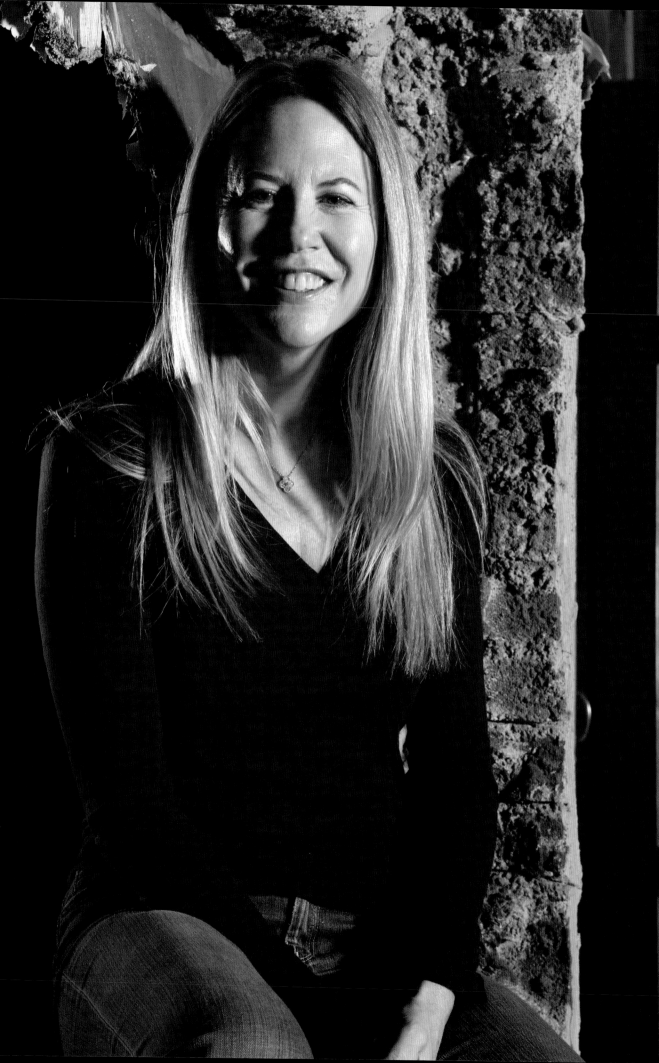

Allegra Clegg

Film Producer
Age at diagnosis, 32
Melanoma, 1993

I never thought about what was happening inside my body until I got cancer. It gave my life a new beginning. I discovered that you have to pay attention to your body. I was only thirty-two years old, so it was a good time to develop new habits and keep them. I started exercising again and eating properly. Within six months, my blood work was already better.

It's important to take control of your body. For me, I took charge of my body in an alternative sense. My philosophy is that you need both Western medicine and alternative help. I need to have good nutrition, learn how my body reacts to different foods, and have complete body awareness, but I also want to regularly see my blood work reports. The doctor said I'm now like a twenty-three-year-old on the inside.

> *I realized that to get healthy, I had to make changes.*

For me, it helps when I talk about it. If you let out the negative, positive things come back. And in turn, it helps others when I share what I have learned. My mother had ovarian cancer a couple of years ago. She is eighty-nine and now back to being very active teaching ballet. Her blood tests are completely cancer-free.

Cancer was a gift because it was a wake-up call to change my life. It was a sign saying, "You've got to get healthy." I realized that to get healthy, I had to make changes.

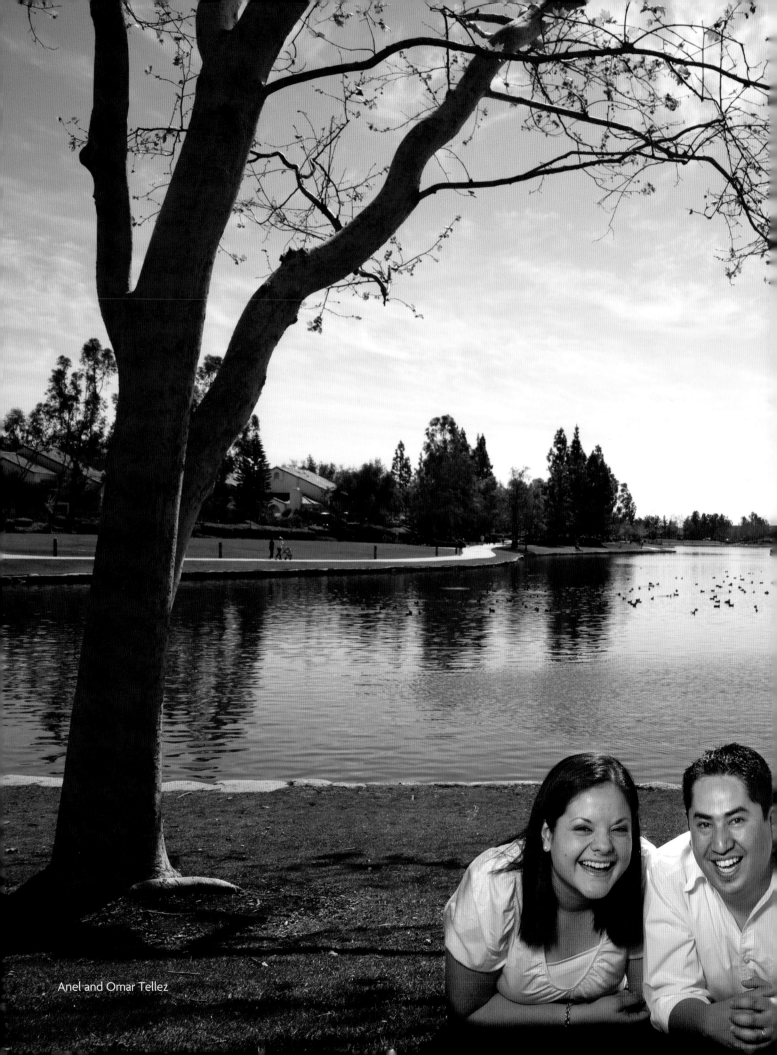

Anel and Omar Tellez

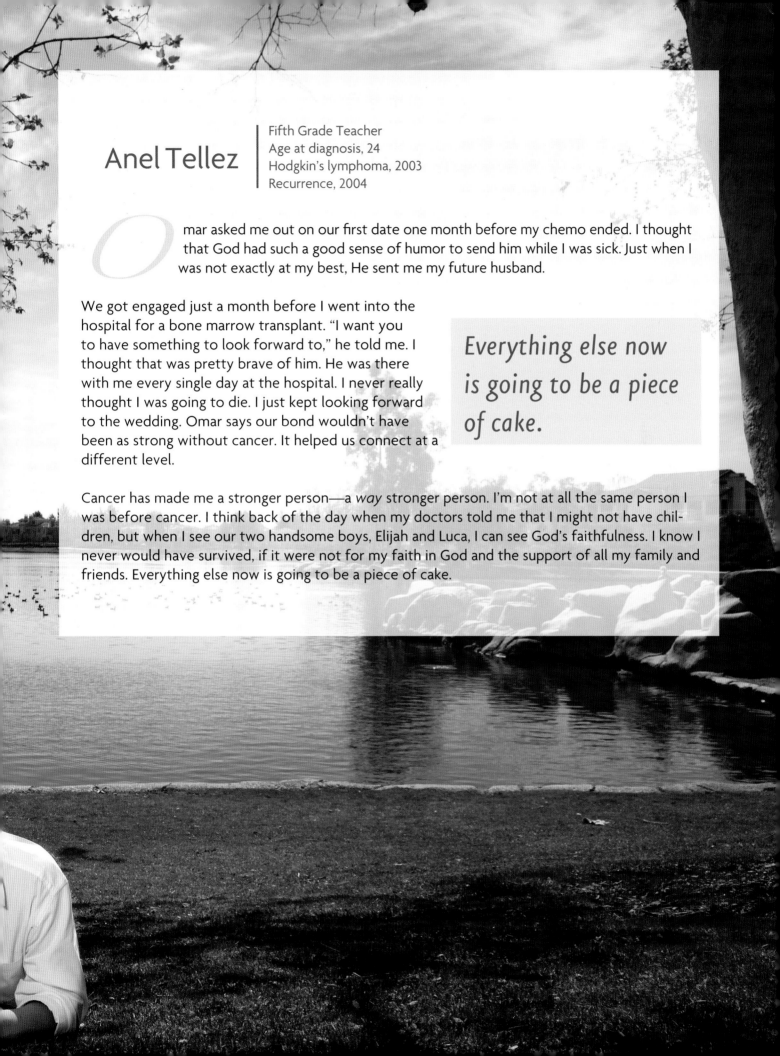

Anel Tellez

Fifth Grade Teacher
Age at diagnosis, 24
Hodgkin's lymphoma, 2003
Recurrence, 2004

Omar asked me out on our first date one month before my chemo ended. I thought that God had such a good sense of humor to send him while I was sick. Just when I was not exactly at my best, He sent me my future husband.

We got engaged just a month before I went into the hospital for a bone marrow transplant. "I want you to have something to look forward to," he told me. I thought that was pretty brave of him. He was there with me every single day at the hospital. I never really thought I was going to die. I just kept looking forward to the wedding. Omar says our bond wouldn't have been as strong without cancer. It helped us connect at a different level.

Everything else now is going to be a piece of cake.

Cancer has made me a stronger person—a *way* stronger person. I'm not at all the same person I was before cancer. I think back of the day when my doctors told me that I might not have children, but when I see our two handsome boys, Elijah and Luca, I can see God's faithfulness. I know I never would have survived, if it were not for my faith in God and the support of all my family and friends. Everything else now is going to be a piece of cake.

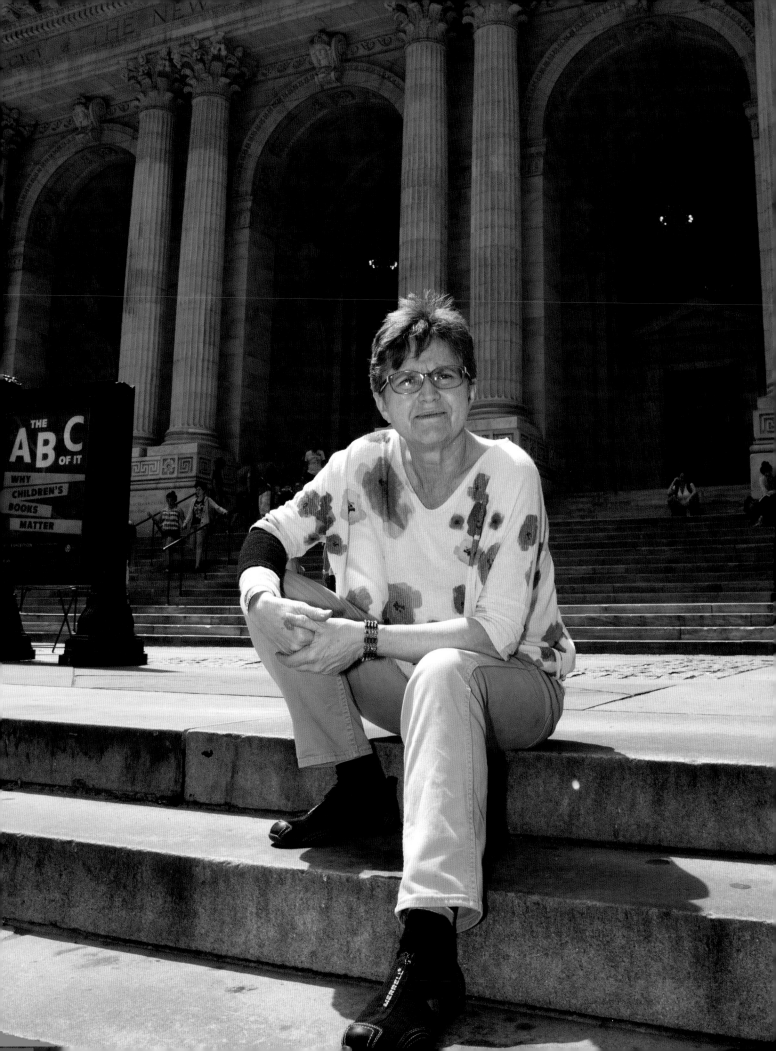

Ann Fonfa

Founder, Annie Appleseed Project
Age at first diagnosis, 44
Breast cancer, 1993, 1995, 1997

They told me I had cancer on a Thursday and scheduled surgery for the next Monday. In my head, that meant it was horrible. It was especially scary because I didn't know anyone who had ever had cancer and lived.

The night before surgery, a complete stranger called me and said she was a ten-year survivor of breast cancer. She saved my life in that moment.

The day after a lumpectomy and the removal of eighteen lymph nodes, I found out I had lymphedema. I had a serious discussion with the doctor about the need for clear and honest conversations before surgery to inform patients about possible outcomes. I didn't realize on that day in 1993 that I was just beginning a life of patient advocacy.

When they told me that I needed chemotherapy, I tried to explain my aversion to chemicals, but the doctor told me it didn't matter. I refused the treatment because I knew the tumor was slow growing and chemo would have no effect and I was seriously chemically sensitive. He thought I was crazy.

I did a lot of reading and research and had a wonderful friend who began treating me with acupuncture. We formed a group around my experience and called it the Whole Health Study Group. With the group's assistance, I was able to promote mind, body, spirit, and health for many others. Our brain controls every cell in our bodies. I wanted to help others access that idea and make a difference in their lives. My husband was with me the entire journey. He supported me in all of my research and in every decision.

> *No one dies from exercising, eating fruits and vegetables, or juicing.*

Two years later, I found a lump. My new surgeon said it was nothing, but the technician suggested I get a biopsy. After they found cancer again, in the exact same spot, the doctor suggested a mastectomy. I had been an antinuclear advocate earlier in my life, and now they wanted to radiate and operate. I refused it all and opted for another lumpectomy. I then went to Canada and researched alternative treatments for healing.

Soon after that, I found six more lumps. Cancer was showing up all over the left breast. Once again, they told me I had to have a mastectomy. This time, I agreed. One year later, when my other breast developed pre-cancer symptoms, I said, "Let's take it off."

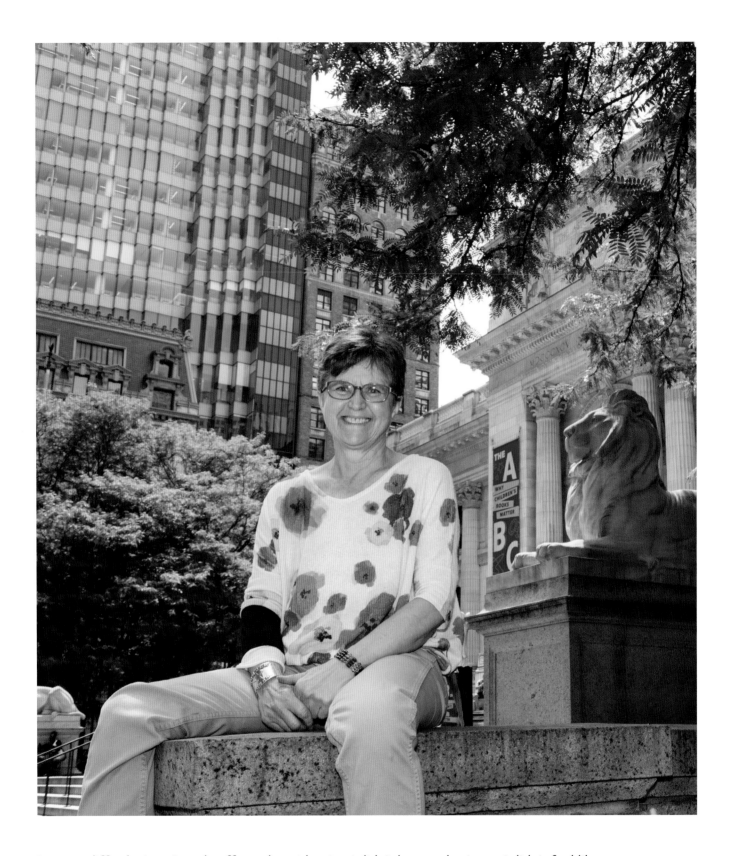

It was a difficult time. It truly affected my identity. I didn't know who I was. I didn't feel like a woman any more. One day, as I was walking down the street in New York City, a gay man said to me, "Great bod!" That comment completely changed my attitude and cured me of all my self-doubt. It's amazing how a simple compliment can change a life.

My path now became to raise awareness. I wrote a sixty-five-page presentation about alternative treatments and took it to the National Breast Cancer Coalition. I started using the name Annie Appleseed Project and posed the question at a medical conference about the use of antioxidants with chemotherapy. I continued posing that question at conferences for the next five years and advocating the use of complementary and integrative treatments.

No one dies from exercising, eating fruits and vegetables, or juicing.

Exercise and diet are important. Annie Appleseed Project's concept is that it all works together in treatment. Healthy behaviors will help heal. Eat one more fruit and one more vegetable every day. Take a walk. Take seven deep breaths before treatment and every night before bedtime. And then relax and enjoy life.

In 1997, when they told me I had stage 4 cancer, it had no meaning to me. I could have suffered, but instead I have used all this time to live life, be happy, and try to help others do the same, which is what I believe brings true happiness. All those corny posters are true. Today is the only day we have.

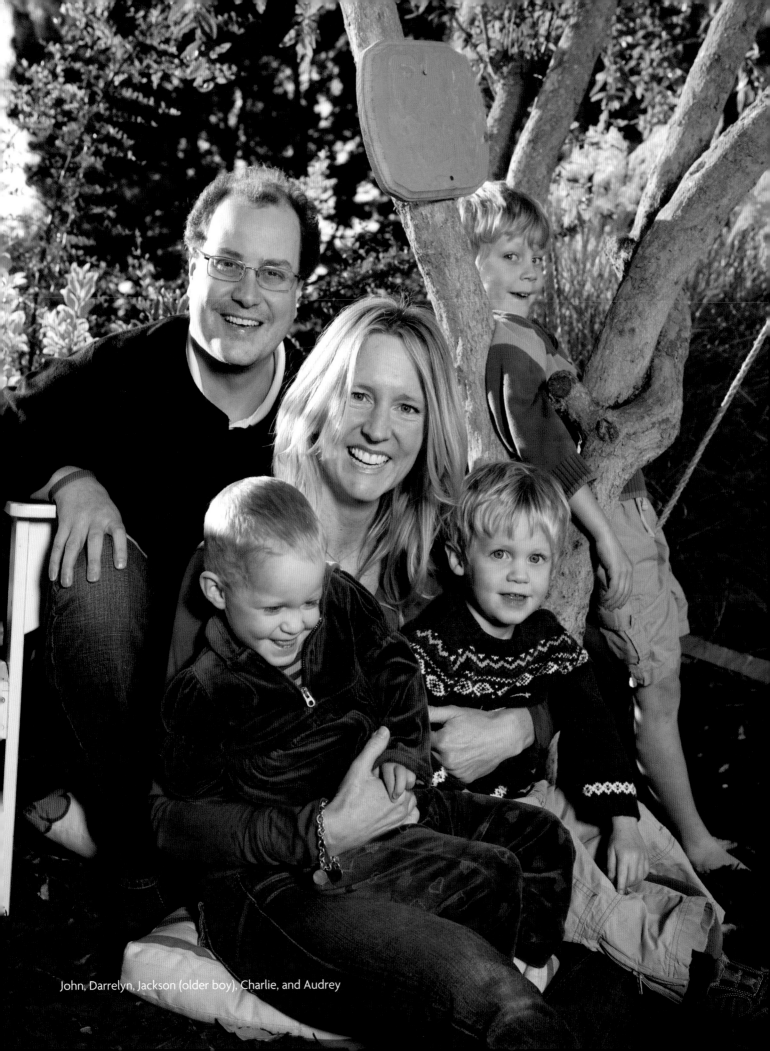

John, Darrelyn, Jackson (older boy), Charlie, and Audrey

Audrey Orr | Age at diagnosis, 22 months
Acute lymphoblastic leukemia (ALL), 2008

*D*ARRELYN, AUDREY'S MOTHER: I think it is so amazing to put stories like ours out there. It's good for all our souls to celebrate the triumphs, but we also need to mourn and grieve for the challenges we fail, so the healing process can begin.

Our experience with Audrey and her leukemia, *our* leukemia really, was life-changing. I wouldn't wish it on anybody, but feel like it was a gift that opened our eyes to so many things. Audrey finished treatment on May 28, 2010, about two years after diagnosis.

She went through so much: countless doctors' appointments, days spent at the hospital hooked up to IVs pumping chemo drugs into her veins, and a couple of unexpected hospital stays due to fever and unexplained infections. She had to take so many different medicines at home every day and even some in the middle of the night.

Every three months throughout treatment she would spend a day at the hospital to undergo an LP— lumbar puncture. They would inject different chemotherapy medicines into her spine and test her spinal fluid. That was the absolute hardest part for me. I was right next to her for every single procedure, and I absolutely hated to see her little body go through all that.

But . . . the reward was her life. No small thing, right? Audrey was so strong and amazing throughout the entire course of her treatment. I will forever remember the day Dr. Finklestein, her primary oncologist, told us Audrey was cancer-free and *done* with treatment.

Today she is a happy, healthy, vibrant seven-year-old second grader, who is surviving and thriving.

We talk and are very open about her leukemia and what we *all* went through. Me, Johnny, and her brothers, Jackson and Charlie. She endured all the physical challenges of treatment, but we all endured the emotional process together. We talk about it but don't dwell on it. We ultimately have no control over what's next, and we can't change things already lost.

> *Cancer can tear families apart, but, for our family, it has centered us.*

I now can truly stop and look back (not dwell) on what we've been through and really appreciate what we have today, right now, at this very moment. I cherish my family with all my heart. They all fill me with a bounty of strength and love that is immeasurable.

JOHN, AUDREY'S FATHER: When you're an adult, there is so much emotion and suffering that goes with having cancer. It can seem like a death sentence. But when you're two years old, you have no idea what's going on. Perhaps that lack of awareness is why young kids often seem to handle it better.

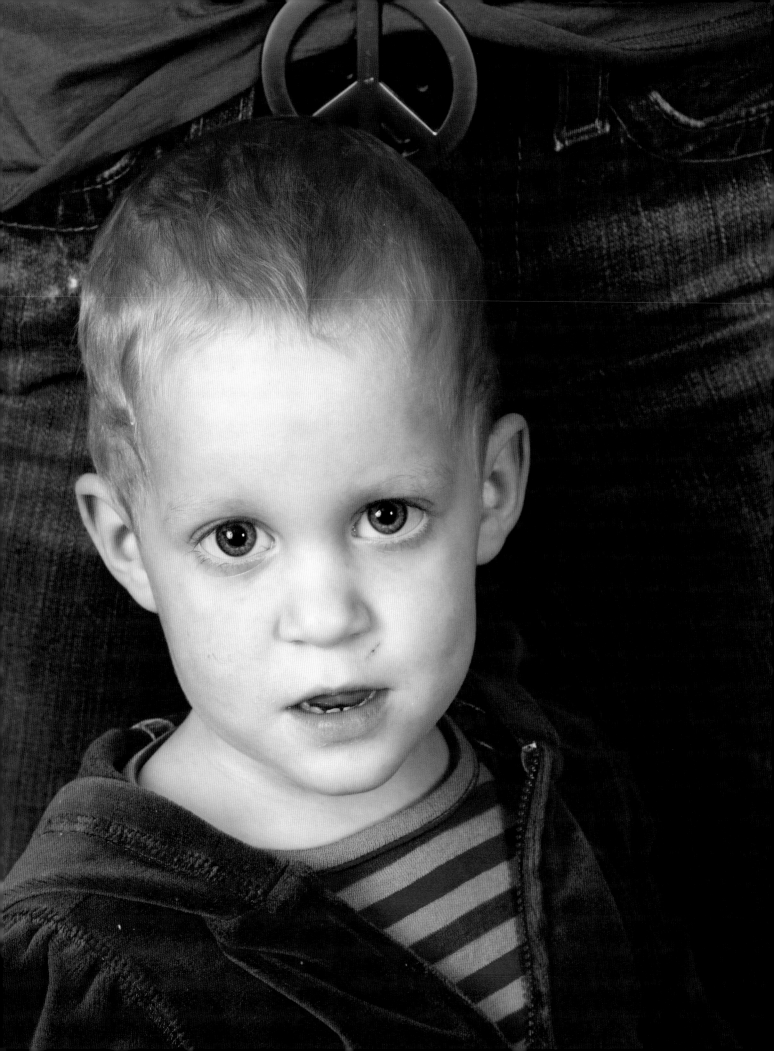

Audrey has made us all stronger. We had to work together as a team. While she was in the hospital, we had to care for two other children at home. The drama absolutely brought us closer together. And it put so much into perspective.

Audrey's doctor told us that, for many families, the diagnosis is like being punched between the eyes. And getting back to health is like hiking up a mountain. There will be steep grades and obstacles along the way, but the goal is to reach the top of the mountain. This became a mantra for our family. Cancer can tear families apart, but, for our family, it has centered us.

We are focused on the goal, the mountaintop. In a very real way—and it may be difficult to understand—we feel fortunate.

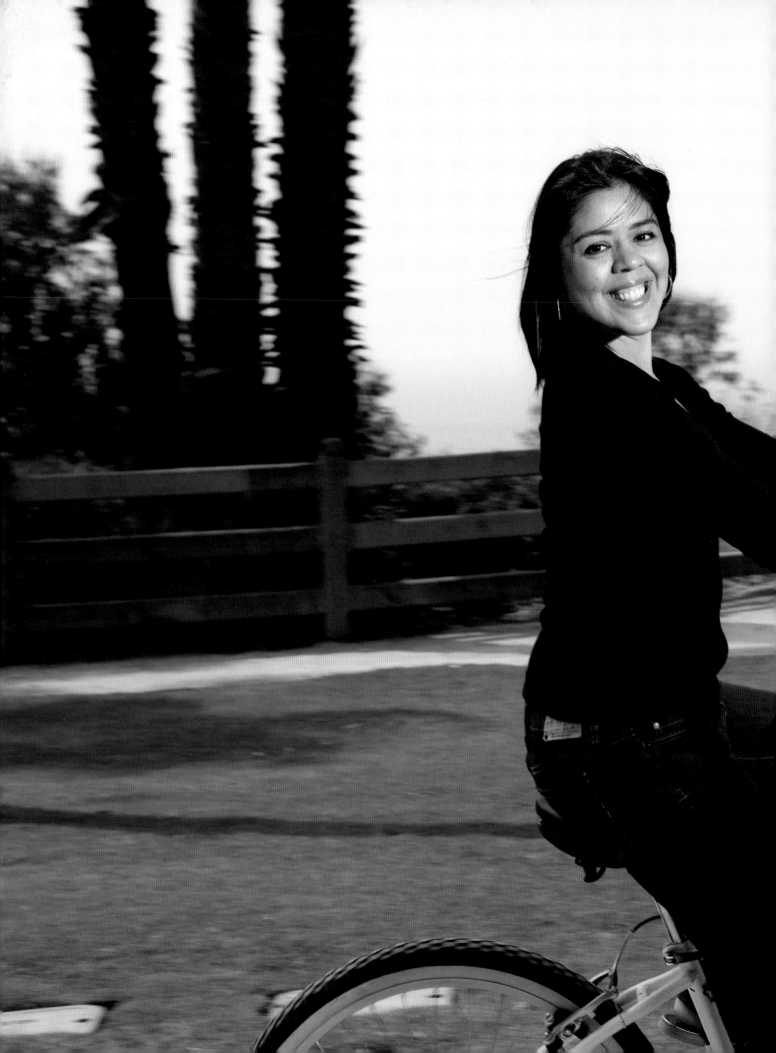

Aurora Avila

Endoscopy Technician, Surgical Center Physician's Assistant
Age at diagnosis, 31
Breast cancer, 2005

I was thirty-one years old, five months into my marriage, and in the first trimester of a pregnancy that I had to terminate. Then came chemotherapy, then surgery, then radiation. And in the middle of it all, I had an emergency appendectomy. A year later I separated from my husband. The entire experience was an awakening for sure.

Cancer forced me to get to know myself deeply, and it forced a spiritual growth that I had never imagined or expected. When you are looking at yourself in the mirror, completely nude without even a strand of hair on your head, you have no choice but to see the real you.

After going through something like this, there is never a "normal" again. There is only a "better." It would be easier to have a normal life, but I don't think I would ever want that. I call it an awakening. Why would I want to go back to sleep? My life is so much better because of everything I went through. Even if I could wave a magic wand and take it all away, I would never do that.

Cancer itself is not a gift, but the lessons you learn as a result of the experience are the gifts.

I feel like it will always be my greatest accomplishment—not just to survive cancer, but to do so without anger or resentment.

I chose to thrive rather than just survive. That is *the* choice.

> *Cancer itself is not a gift, but the lessons you learn as a result of the experience are the gifts.*

> *I chose to thrive rather than just survive. That is the choice.*

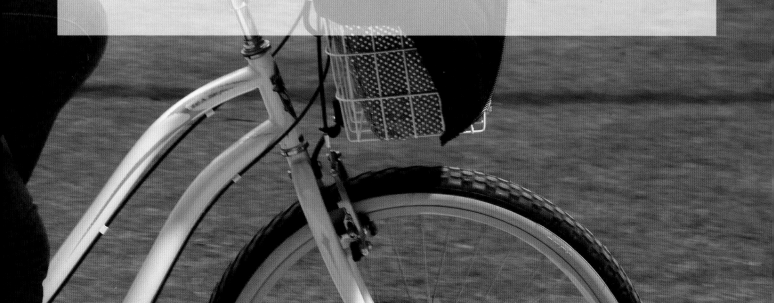

Barbie Zolla
Children's Services Worker and Realtor
Age at diagnosis, 67
Pancreatic cancer, 2007

Marshall Zolla
Attorney
Age at first diagnosis, 69
Prostate cancer, 2008
Kidney cancer, 2009

BARBIE: I had never been sick a day in my life. I had never even taken a sick day at work. So it was a shock when I got my diagnosis. But I was not going to let it change who I am. I'm a very determined person. Nothing stops me. If I want to do something, I do it, no matter what.

Every day I have an agenda, and I schedule lunch with someone to keep me from sitting home feeling sorry for myself. I just keep my mind off of it. Some people tell me I am in denial, but for me it's a coping mechanism. This is a choice to live a normal life, not a denial.

My family thought I needed a psychiatrist, but he kept telling me about the severity of cancer. I didn't want to hear that. That makes me feel down, and I want to feel up. I'm not going to RSVP to the pity party.

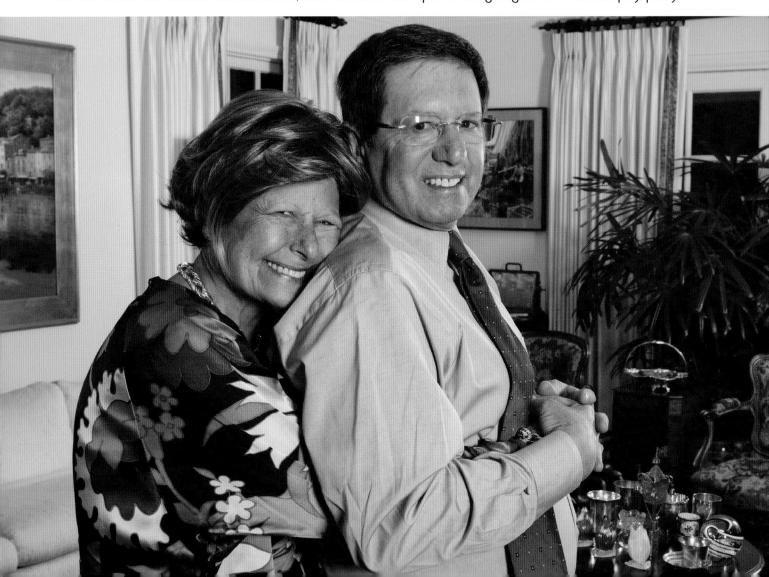

When Marshall got cancer too, I felt the same way about him. I knew he'd get through it. I wasn't going to feel sorry for him either.

MARSHALL: That's right. I sure didn't get much sympathy from her. Barbie has been an inspiration to me and to all of our friends because of her strength.

One night she had a very high fever. I told her to get up and get dressed to go to the emergency room, or else I was calling 911. She refused to get up. A few minutes later when there were five paramedics in our bedroom, she told them to leave. She finally gave up and went with me to the hospital. I felt bad, but I couldn't let her strength get in the way of her healing. We learned later that we had probably saved her life.

And then when I got sick, it became physically and emotionally difficult to be a good caregiver to Barbie. That was hard for me.

BARBIE: A few other things also have truly helped.

We laugh a lot. Humor is very important.

And I don't judge others. Everyone is important. Even if they say something inappropriate, I know they mean well.

MARSHALL: Barbie wanted to start planning our fortieth wedding anniversary six months early, and quite frankly, I wasn't sure she would still be here. We recently celebrated the milestone with a dinner dance, and she was lovely. I ended my toast with a reference to Moses' farewell address in the Bible. After forty years, he tells his people that he could not have shouldered his burdens alone. It was a very appropriate story for us, because in our forty years, we have not had to shoulder our burdens alone. We were surrounded with the love, strength, and compassion of all our friends in the room that night.

> *I'm not going to RSVP to the pity party.*

> *We laugh a lot. Humor is very important.*

2014 Update

Marshall: In January 2010 I was in the UCLA Medical Center for a major operation to remove a malignant tumor in my left kidney. The next morning, while I was still heavily sedated, Barbie went in for a chemotherapy treatment, suffered a stroke, and passed away in the same hospital. Our daughter was eight months pregnant. Six weeks later, our first grandchild was born. Five months later, I was invited to study for a week at the Shalom Hartman Institute in Jerusalem and then spent a week in the desert. I came back renewed and healed. Two years later, I met someone and fell in love again.

Beth Hersh Goldsmith

Executive Director, Craig H. Neilsen Foundation
Age at diagnosis, 54
Appendiceal cancer, 2011
Recurrence, April 2013

I knew something was wrong when I tried on a dress that I planned to wear to a wedding. It was so tight that I couldn't fit into it.

How could this be? I was in great physical condition. My husband, Gordy, and I were training to go biking in the hills of Italy. I bought another dress a size larger but, two days later, that one didn't fit either.

On Monday, Memorial Day, I went on a thirty-mile ride in the hills. On Tuesday, I called my doctor and said, "You know what? I think I have cancer." I suggested a complete blood count and two cancer marker tests, and he agreed.

Two days later, he called and told me that my blood counts were fine. When I asked about the markers, he cursed and admitted, "They lost that tube of blood. They didn't do the markers."

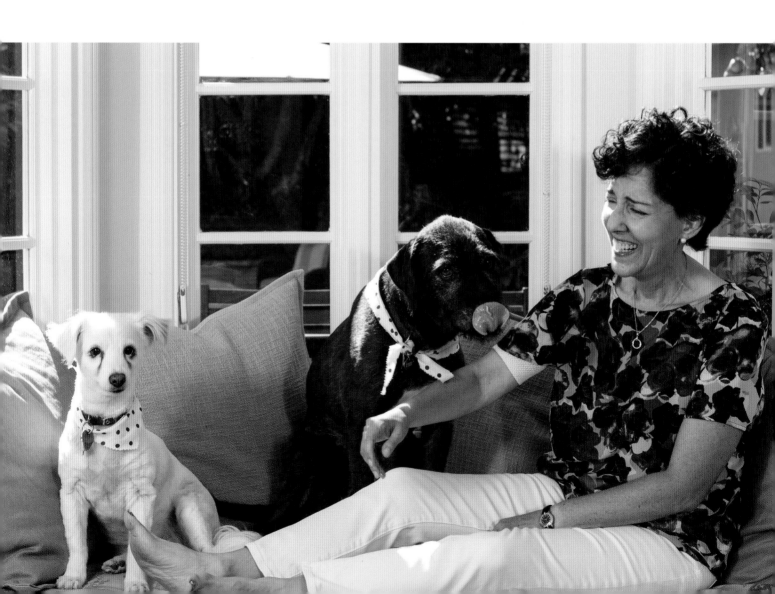

When I returned from a business trip six days later, I looked five months pregnant. On a Friday afternoon, an ultrasound and scan confirmed my suspicions.

My doctor, a good friend, was crying when he came to see me with the scan results. I said, "Crap. This is one time I wish I was wrong."

I asked a friend (and physician) at City of Hope, "If we bring you the CD with my scan, can you pop it into your computer and tell me what I have?" He said that it wasn't quite that easy but agreed to go in on Sunday. He said he would bring in the best radiologist and they would stay until they figured it out.

Turns out I have one of the world's rarest cancers. It started in my appendix and had been growing for three to five years. The tumors are tough to spot because they hide in mucin, a gel. Typically, there are no solid tumors.

On Monday morning, I went to COH for eight hours of tests and consultations. Two days later, I was on the operating table for twelve hours. They tried to save what they could but had to remove six organs. Then they poured heated chemo into my belly and gently rocked me back and forth for ninety minutes to spread the chemo.

They drained it, closed me up and put me into a coma for a few days. When I woke up, Gordy asked if I wanted anything. I had a ventilator and was frustrated because I tried to communicate that I wanted KPCC (the local public radio station), but they thought I wanted KFC. Gordy told the doctor, "We've been together for thirty-two years, and I've never seen her eat fried chicken."

My blood pressure shot way up because they couldn't figure out what I wanted. The doctor put me back to "sleep" for twenty-four more hours to calm me down.

Our daughter Aliza was the one who figured out that I wanted to listen to KPCC. It seems she knew me better than anyone.

After the surgery I did twelve rounds of chemo and was technically in remission. After my one-year anniversary, it reared its ugly head again.

This time, I had a laparoscopy at MD Anderson and was scheduled to remove the new cancer in Houston two months later. After another scan the day before the scheduled surgery, the

Cancer has taught me that I no longer have control of my disease or my destiny.

surgeon came in and apologized, "Sorry I'm late, but I've been talking to your COH doctors. The scan shows new cancer, both the gel and a solid tumor." They decided to remove the tumor.

The procedure was very tricky but the team at MD Anderson thought all was well. I recovered, flew to Los Angeles and four days later, I passed out; the surgery had caused a hematoma (internal bleeding), and a complete bowel obstruction. After eight days in the hospital, I was fed TPN (liquid nutrition) through a PICC line for a month before I was strong enough to start chemo.

After six rounds, we found the chemo had done nothing. I consulted with specialists around the country, and the unanimous recommendation was to add Avastin, a monoclonal antibody that stops the blood supply to the tumors. We tried it and, remarkably, my markers have come way down.

Through all of this, I'm still amazed at the support from family and friends. My husband has been the researcher par excellence. He's never missed a doctor's appointment. Our daughter and son, Noah, took turns staying in the hospital with me every single night after my surgeries. And our friends brought us meals for nine months, four nights a week.

My markers are still not in the normal range. God willing, we can keep this cancer at bay but it's very aggressive. I'm holding my breath until the next scan.

And while I wait, I realize I have no control over my situation. For a control-freak, that's very difficult. As an Executive Director for the past twenty-seven years, I was always in control. Even my home healthcare nurse commented that I'm her only patient in control of all of the supplies that I need for my care. Cancer has taught me that I no longer have control of my disease or my destiny.

And so I enjoy each day and try to see the good in everything.

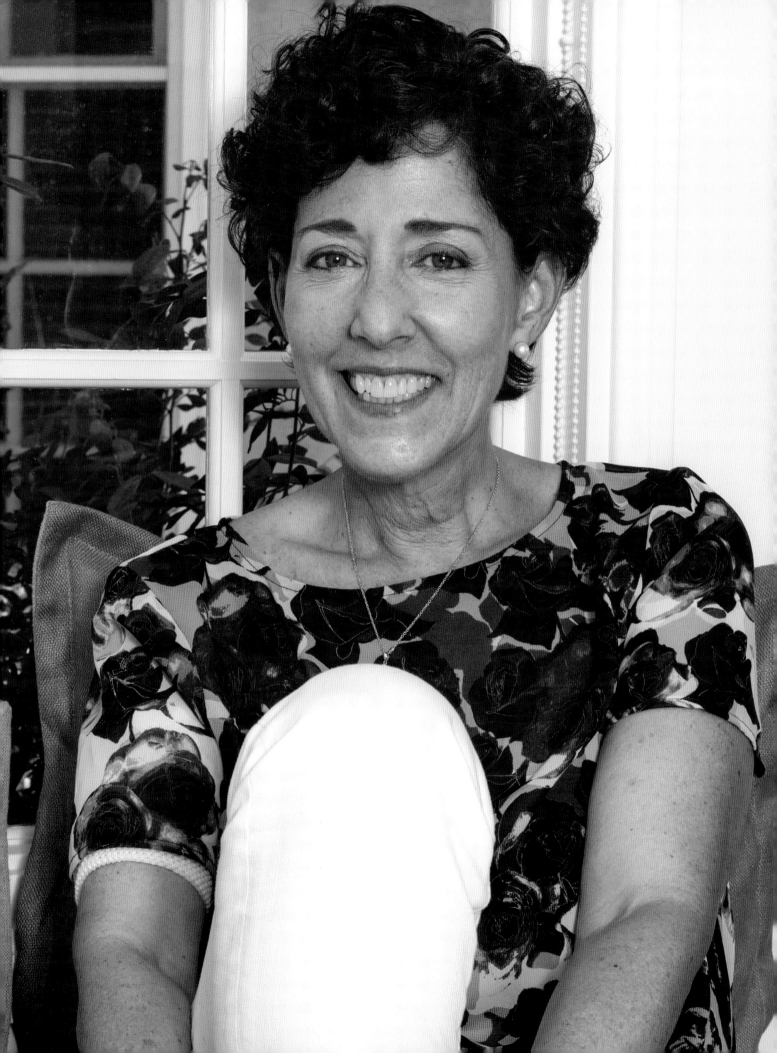

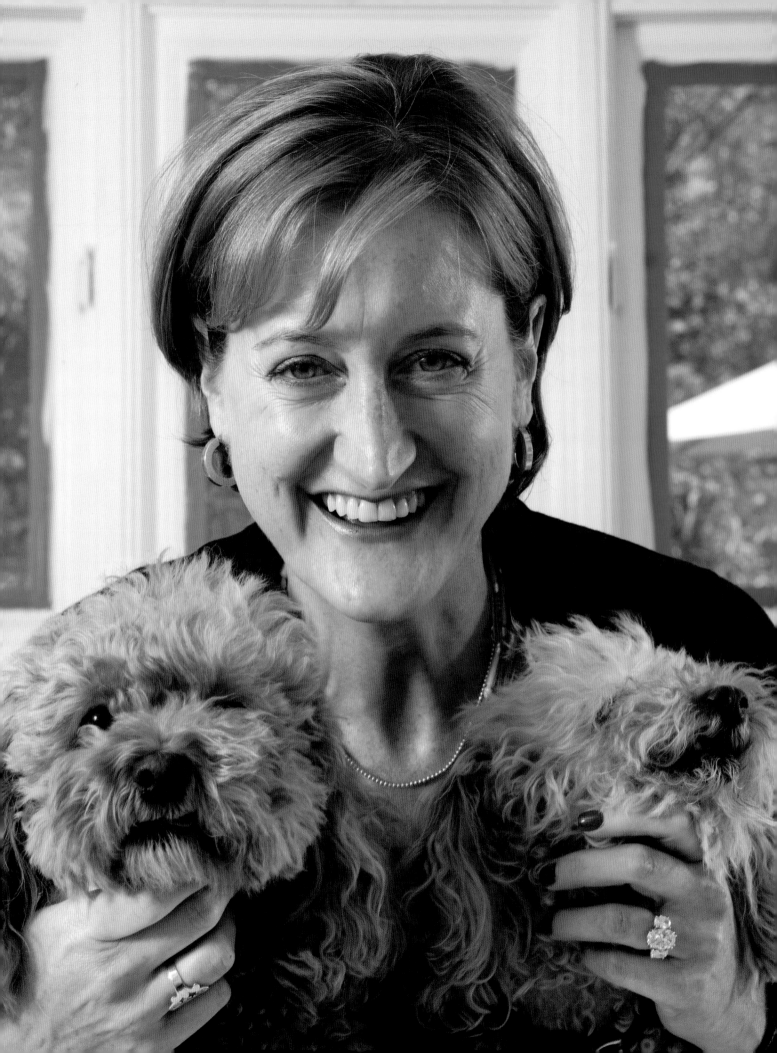

Betsy Leder

Interior Designer
Age at diagnosis, 24
Hodgkin's lymphoma, stage 2, 1984

When I was young I was always anxious about getting sick. Then I did get sick. People told me that it was the best kind of cancer to have if you have to have cancer. Since I was living in a small town in Indiana, where they didn't have radiation machines, I moved in with my brother in Louisville, Kentucky.

At the time, I really didn't think there was any residual emotional impact. But the following summer when I led a group of college kids to Israel, we were singing and I suddenly became overwhelmed with emotion. I ran from the building and started sobbing. I couldn't stop. It all came out.

I volunteer in the ER at a hospital once a week. Whenever I see someone coming in who is being treated for cancer, some of the fear returns. It's less intense than it used to be, but it's there.

I met my husband-to-be a short time after my treatments. My hair still had gray tips from the radiation. He told me to cut my hair short and be proud of who and what I was. Ten days later, we were engaged.

I've become very concerned now about diet and nutrition. I try to eat extremely healthy foods. I hate to drive my kids crazy with my eating habits, but they are my kids.

. . . the time spent worrying is time wasted.

I still have a nagging fear of getting cancer again. I think a certain degree of anxiety is inevitable. But I have also learned that the time spent worrying is time wasted. So I try to teach my children that fear need not be a part of their healthy emotional diet.

Mostly I've learned that if you want to do something, don't be afraid . . . just do it.

Mostly I've learned that if you want to do something, don't be afraid . . . just do it.

Beverlye Hyman Fead

Artist, Poet
Age at first diagnosis, 57
Uterine lining cancer, 1991
Uterine stromal sarcoma, stage 4, 2003

C ells from my first cancer had drifted into my abdomen and were growing there until the doctors found them twelve years later. I was given two months to live, and yet I felt fine except for some stomach pains. I had been working out, eating right, and living well, so I convinced myself there was nothing wrong with me. Now I realize I was living in denial.

There was some crying and depression during this time, because I didn't know what the outcome would be. Good news from the doctors would take me up, and then bad news would bring me down. I was finally accepted for an experimental treatment of shots and pills. I grabbed at it, rather than take the

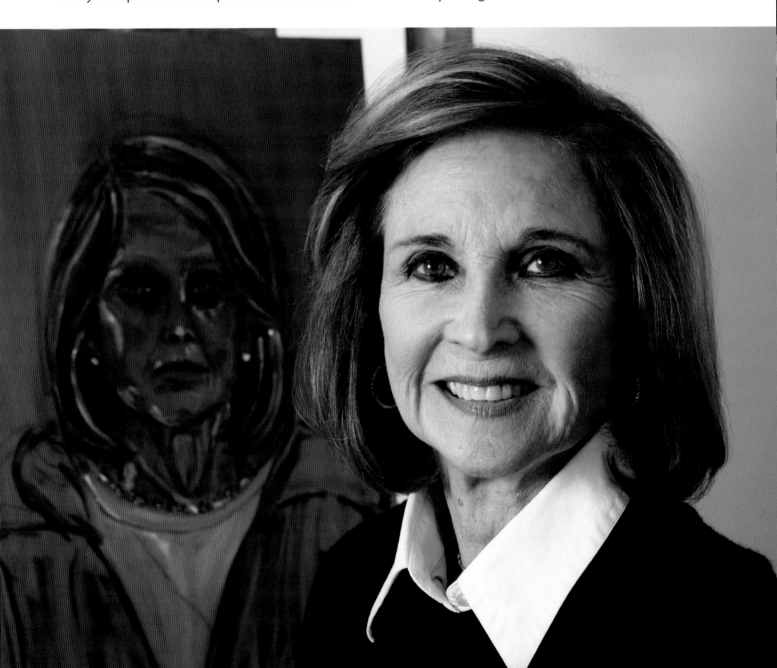

traditional treatment of chemotherapy and an operation. I got my first shot and pill eleven years ago, and I've never looked back. These eleven years have been the most powerful years of my life because I am so passionate about helping other cancer patients. I tell them not to give up when they get their diagnosis.

I speak at high schools, colleges, and cancer centers. I want everyone to know that cancer isn't what it used to be. You no longer just lie down and die. There are so many options now. So many people are living with their cancer today or are even cancer-free. The numbers keep getting better and better. I tell every patient I meet, "You are a co-captain with your doctor. He has hundreds of patients, but you have only one. Be an advocate for yourself."

> *. . . cancer isn't what it used to be. You no longer just lie down and die. There are so many options now.*

Without cancer, my life would not have been as meaningful. I feel so much more purposeful. I feel I have made my life count by helping those I didn't even know. I have written two books. The first one is *I Can Do This: Living with Cancer,* and the second one is a children's book that I wrote with my granddaughter called *Nana, What's Cancer?* I also produced a short documentary called *Stage 4, Living with Cancer.*

I'm going to do as much as I can to help others while I'm here on earth. I may not be able to hike the tall mountains that I used to, but I still play golf, and I walk a lot. I don't take anything for granted. We moved to a new place on the beach and its peacefulness is therapeutic for my creativity, in all forms.

Cancer is a bittersweet thing that happens to you. On every holiday I am sad that it might be my last, and yet I look at life with such gratitude and joy that I'm here to enjoy it with my family.

Beverlye Hyman Fead was awarded the National Profile of Courage Award from the National Sarcoma Society, 2009.

Beverlye Hyman Fead was awarded the National Profile of Courage Award from the National Sarcoma Society, 2009.

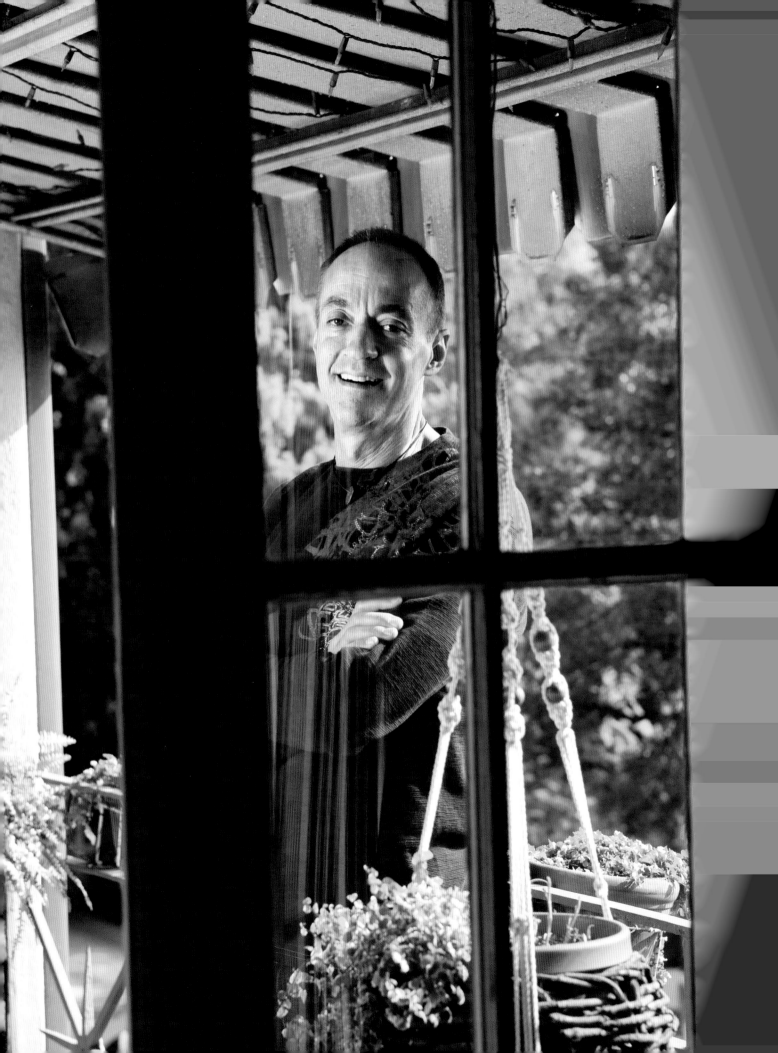

Bill Kavanagh

Program Manager at Cancer Support Community
Age at diagnosis, 53
Hodgkin's lymphoma, stage 4, 2008

I have been HIV positive for twenty-nine years. Back then, it was a death sentence. They gave me five years at the most. So I've already been through the "gonna-die" routine. Once again, though, my world was slammed into harsh reality and sudden introspection.

The oncologist told me on December 24 that I had cancer. I remember saying to him, "Merry Christmas to you, too. Sorry I didn't get you anything." But then I told him immediately that I have learned several times in life that our biggest challenges always present us with our most rewarding gifts. As it turns out, it was the greatest Christmas gift I have ever received.

. . . our biggest challenges always present us with our most rewarding gifts.

As odd as it sounds, one of the most valuable gifts was the inability to do anything. Much of the time during chemo, all I could do was think and write. Most people are never given the incredible gift of forced reflection. You can do nothing but sit and think about what is important. You can choose to think about the bad or you can choose to focus on the good, and celebrate all the great things and people that surround you. I thought about the future.

My cousin's son is twenty years old and was visiting me recently with his girlfriend. They asked my advice for two young people about to start their lives. I told them not to be afraid to take risks. Jumping off the cliff is the only way to learn to fly. Then they told me that they were so excited about the future. They have no idea how profound that was for me. They made me realize that age has no bearing on our level of excitement about our future. Cancer gave me a new future just as if I were twenty again.

I attended Antioch University and graduated in 2012 with my master's in clinical psychology. I now work at the Cancer Support Community, Benjamin Center, facilitating support groups for people with cancer and their caregivers. If ever there was a purpose for getting cancer, I have found it. When I told my oncologist on Christmas Eve, 2007, that I looked forward to discovering the blessings of my diagnosis, I never could have imagined such a dramatic change toward an impactful life.

I know one thing for sure . . . I'm willing to jump. I want to fly.

I know one thing for sure . . . I'm willing to jump. I want to fly.

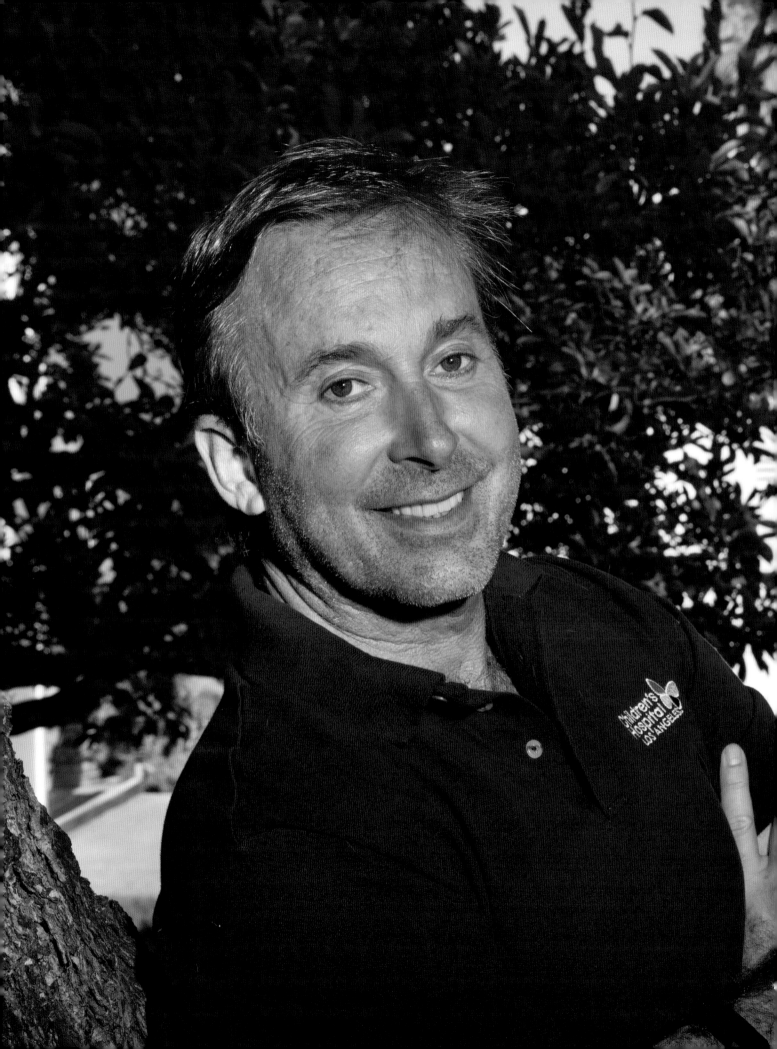

Bill Kenny

Registered Nurse, Children's Hospital Los Angeles
Age at first diagnosis, 30
Testicular cancer, 1990, 1993

I was thirty when I was diagnosed with cancer in my right testicle. The treatment that was recommended, and that I followed, was to have an orchiectomy followed up with radiation therapy for six weeks on my abdomen.

Three years later, I was having some general fatigue. I knew something was wrong, but it never occurred to me that it was cancer again. Testicular cancer in more than one testicle is very rare, but this was a much more aggressive cell type. The surgeon removed the lymph nodes behind my stomach and recommended follow-up chemotherapy. That was tough news and I took it very hard.

Learning that I could never have children was somewhat depressing. Many men have told me that they would rather die than lose their testicles. It was mind boggling to hear that. I was only thirty-three years old, I had survived cancer twice, and I was alive.

I laughingly told my mom, "Compared to junior high, cancer was easy." It was a joke, but at the same time, felt true. I had felt alone in junior high, but with cancer, everyone jumped in to help. I was well cared for. Ironically, I have very good memories of my time with cancer. At that young age, I got to experience real love.

After cancer, I was ill prepared when the realities of life kicked in. That's why the Cancer Support Community group was such a godsend. The community told me that the moment I was diagnosed, I became a cancer survivor. I liked that way of thinking. I also discovered that most everyone in my group experienced their own lessons of love.

At the time, I was a sitcom-writer and producer. Most people think that life in TV is glamorous and that I was living a dream. But, for me, it was extremely stressful. I faced constant deadlines and always had to prove myself. During my treatments, I contemplated a different future; cancer allowed me to explore the possibility of a new path. I had watched the doctors and nurses every day, and I saw how they faced real life with intimate, personal conversations. My job felt superficial by comparison.

Over the next few years, I changed my priorities and my life. When I went back to school for nursing, my friends thought I was crazy. But now as an RN at Children's Hospital in Los Angeles, some of these same friends tell me they wish they

> *Don't wait until you get cancer to change your life.*

had the courage to do what I did. My answer to them is simple. Don't wait until you get cancer to change your life. Cancer taught me to reevaluate my priorities and to be captain of my own ship. I consciously tried to find ways to reduce stress and anxiety. I told myself I wanted to commit to traveling more. Still to this day, I take a big trip every year. I set aside part of my budget to fulfill that priority, which is so important to me.

I've now been at Children's Hospital for nine years, and every day I experience children who are facing challenges that might overwhelm you or me. But these kids still laugh, play, and get excited about balloons and ice cream. They remind me that no matter what life brings, there's always something to get excited about.

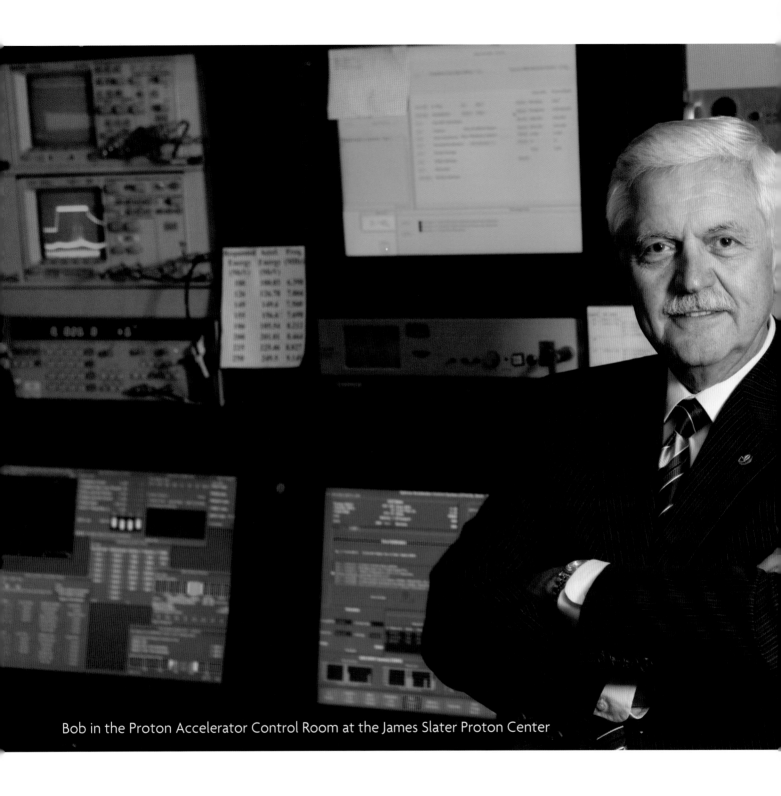

Bob in the Proton Accelerator Control Room at the James Slater Proton Center

When I look back, the best things that ever happened to me were meeting my wife, having my kids, and getting prostate cancer.

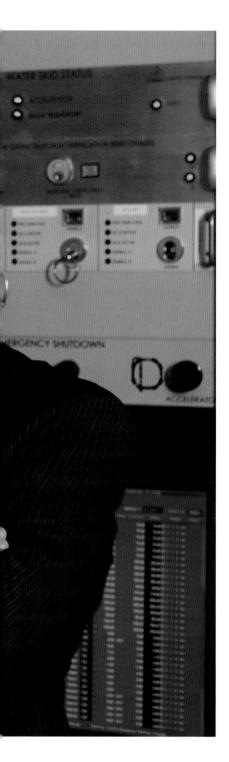

Bob Marckini | Author, Business Consultant
Age at diagnosis, 57
Prostate cancer, 2000

After my diagnosis, I was confused. With prostate cancer, there are so many types of treatments. You can cook it, cut it, freeze it, or whatever. That's when my education began. I shifted my entire emphasis to interviewing former patients. Because of my business background, I always believed that if you're going to buy a new product and invest a lot of money in it, you should go out and talk to the customers.

I was brought up in a family where you couldn't even use the word *cancer*. So I grew up believing it was a death sentence. When I started doing research and learning more about the disease, I started feeling a little bit more comfortable and in control. And when I discovered proton therapy, I felt a huge weight lifted. Not only do I not have to die, I can come through this intact. I was inspired and energized

But you're not cured when you walk out. Healing is a total process—body, mind, and spirit. Yes, they shoot protons in your prostate, but that is only a small part of the healing. Personally, I went from the shock of terrible news of diagnosis to great treatment to giving back.

At Loma Linda hospital, there is a daily support group. All of us became a close family, so afterward I suggested to other men in the program that we stay in touch and share information. That was the start of a group jokingly referred to as "The Brotherhood of the Balloon" because in proton therapy, they use a rectal balloon to treat you. Our mission is to provide communication, information, and support to each other. When I finished treatment, we had nineteen members in our group. As of 2013, we're now 6,500 people strong, in all fifty states and thirty-five countries.

Prostate cancer gave me a chance to create something out of nothing and to help people through a bad experience. Twenty years ago at a cocktail party someone asked what I would want as an epitaph on my tombstone. I remember my answer was "He made a difference." I hadn't thought about that in many years, but cancer gave me a chance to make a difference in people's lives.

Life is good, playing golf and enjoying my granddaughter. When I look back, the best things that ever happened to me were meeting my wife, having my kids, and getting prostate cancer.

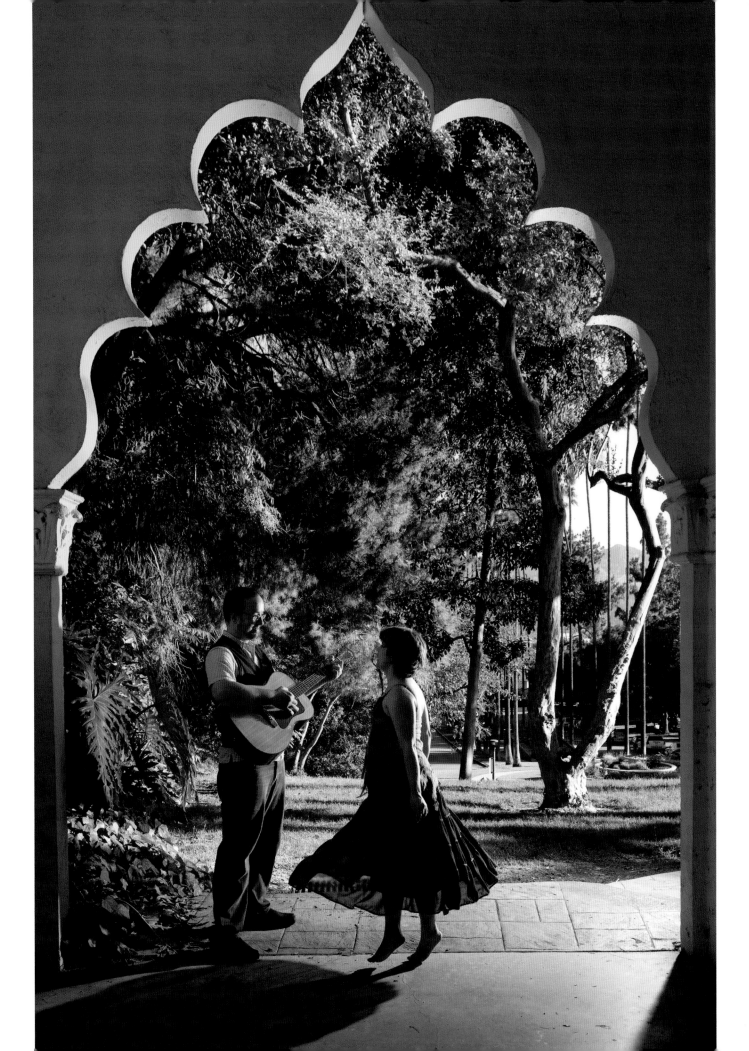

Brandon Schott

Singer, Song Writer, Producer, Musician
Age at diagnosis, 32
Extragonadal germ cell tumor in chest, 2007

Cancer truly was one of the most inspiring events of my life. I saw the best of humanity, and I was left with an incredible perspective for moving forward.

Whether it's cancer or anything else that gets hard in life, there is potential for transformation. I am much calmer now. I've learned that you don't know what you can do until you've tried it. I'm empowered, balanced, and I try to keep things in better perspective. It's okay now not to balance the checkbook, and I can have dirty laundry. I'll just dust off a dirty shirt and do the laundry the next day.

As difficult as it was, cancer gave me a renewed vision of the world. Spirituality, for me, is that force which binds us all together as people. Ultimately when we choose to serve God, we choose to serve that spirit, that common bond that we all share together. The amount of love that surrounded me was beautifully overwhelming. I saw spirituality in action.

I knew the energy wasn't mine to keep. I was just borrowing it for a little while, so I've since aimed to pay it back and help others in return wherever I can. I started bonding with other like-minded artists, community leaders—survivors of one transformation or another—who all wanted to share this love, to celebrate and champion causes close to our hearts. From all of this, I still write songs that seem to pour out of the air. I barely remember writing them. They are gifts from some other plane to help me understand and cope with all the new energy that swirls around me as I continue to live out my cancer story.

> *It's like he's young again without cancer, only better.*

MICHELLE, BRANDON'S WIFE: We have a new faith in each other as well. His cancer gave us a type of rediscovery and renewal. I have a little bit of a crush on him like I did in the beginning. It's like he's young again without cancer, only better.

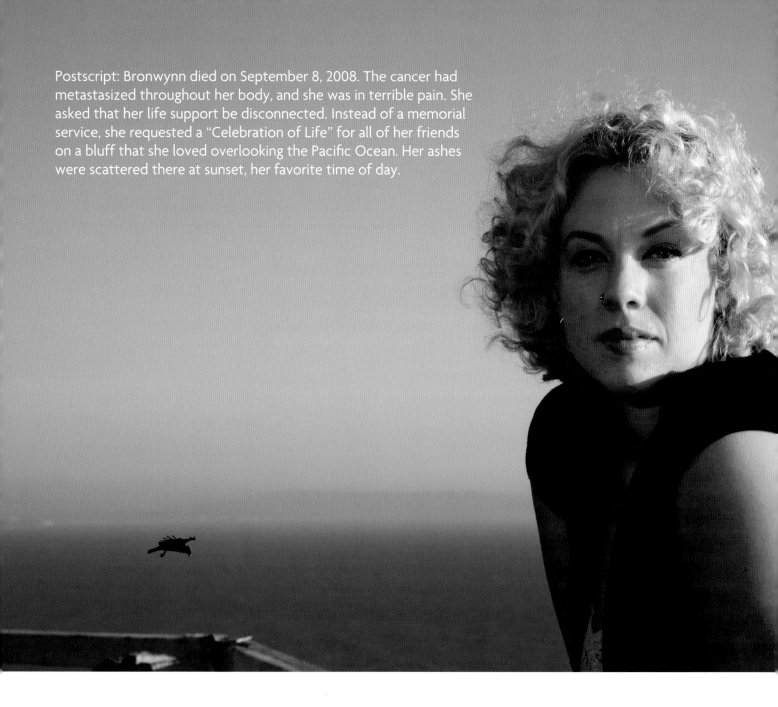

Postscript: Bronwynn died on September 8, 2008. The cancer had metastasized throughout her body, and she was in terrible pain. She asked that her life support be disconnected. Instead of a memorial service, she requested a "Celebration of Life" for all of her friends on a bluff that she loved overlooking the Pacific Ocean. Her ashes were scattered there at sunset, her favorite time of day.

I know now that anything is possible, and I have a sense that something truly amazing is about to happen.

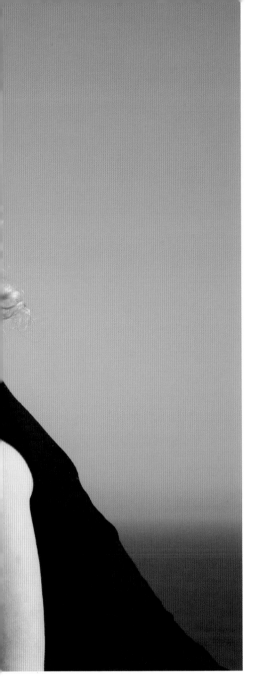

Bronwynn Saifer

Age at diagnosis, 22
Metastatic breast cancer, stage 4,
HER2-positive, 2006

Because I was so young, it took me six months of begging doctors to look at the lump and do a biopsy. I was eventually diagnosed with the most aggressive form of breast cancer.

Before cancer, my life was horrible. I was the unhappiest, most stressed-out, neurotic, worrywart you'd ever want to meet. Life was a struggle from every angle. And the entire time I was growing up, I was obsessed about getting cancer. When I was diagnosed, it was actually a relief because I didn't have to worry any longer that I might get it. Surreal is an understatement.

I always used to live in the past. Now, for the first time in my life, I'm actually living, not just surviving. I know how to be compassionate and gentle with myself. I can avoid a lot of suffering by just allowing my feelings to be what they are.

(After our interview and photography session, Bronwynn sent the following email):

Strange as it may sound, I am actually happy to have been diagnosed with cancer. Happy is the best word I can find. I feel like I am finally becoming the person I've always wanted to be. I have conquered my biggest fear. Although I visit fear, I no longer *live* in it. And that is the greatest joy and freedom I have ever experienced. Cancer has been a catalyst for me to live more fully and to love more deeply. And if one day I do transition from this consciousness to another, I would not want to change a thing. It has been my greatest teacher. For that I am grateful.

Inner peace is something I am able to maintain *at times*. Not *all* times. I cannot honestly say how I would feel on my "death bed." I do not by *any means* want to give anyone the impression that I am floating on clouds all day long, because I fall apart regularly. But that's okay with me. That is the biggest difference between pre- and post-cancer. I know now that anything is possible, and I have a sense that something truly amazing is about to happen.

Carl Douglas Rogers

Communications Consultant/Writer
Age at first diagnosis, 39
Kidney cancer, 1993
Colon cancer, 1997
Prostate cancer, 1998
Metastases 2010, 2012, 2014

Because of a long family history of cancer, it wasn't until my second diagnosis that I developed what I call a "cancer consciousness," taking charge of my health and life.

I quit smoking, changed my diet, and went to a support group. I learned how my attitudes, behavior, and nutrition all play a role in my quality of life. I couldn't do anything about genetics, and I couldn't leave where I lived in Los Angeles, but I could make other significant lifestyle changes.

I joined a weekly cancer support group at the Cancer Support Community in Santa Monica. Its founder, Dr. Howard Benjamin, taught me that "People with cancer who participate in their fight for recovery . . . will improve the quality of their lives and may enhance the possibility of their recovery."

I took those words to heart. I fought for life over cancer and ended up better off because of it. As a patient advocate, I've been honored to serve for several years now on a National Cancer Institute editorial board dealing with complementary and alternative medicine.

I fought for life over cancer and ended up better off because of it.

Even though my prostate cancer has metastasized three different times, making survival more the issue now than recovery—and more medical intervention a reality—I still remain one of those people who believe that cancer is the best thing that ever happened to me.

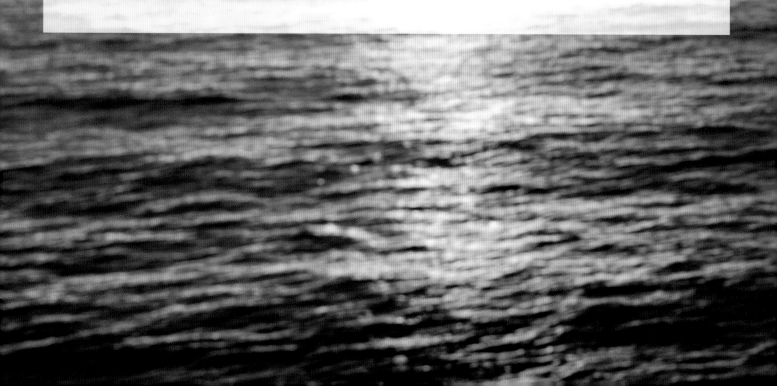

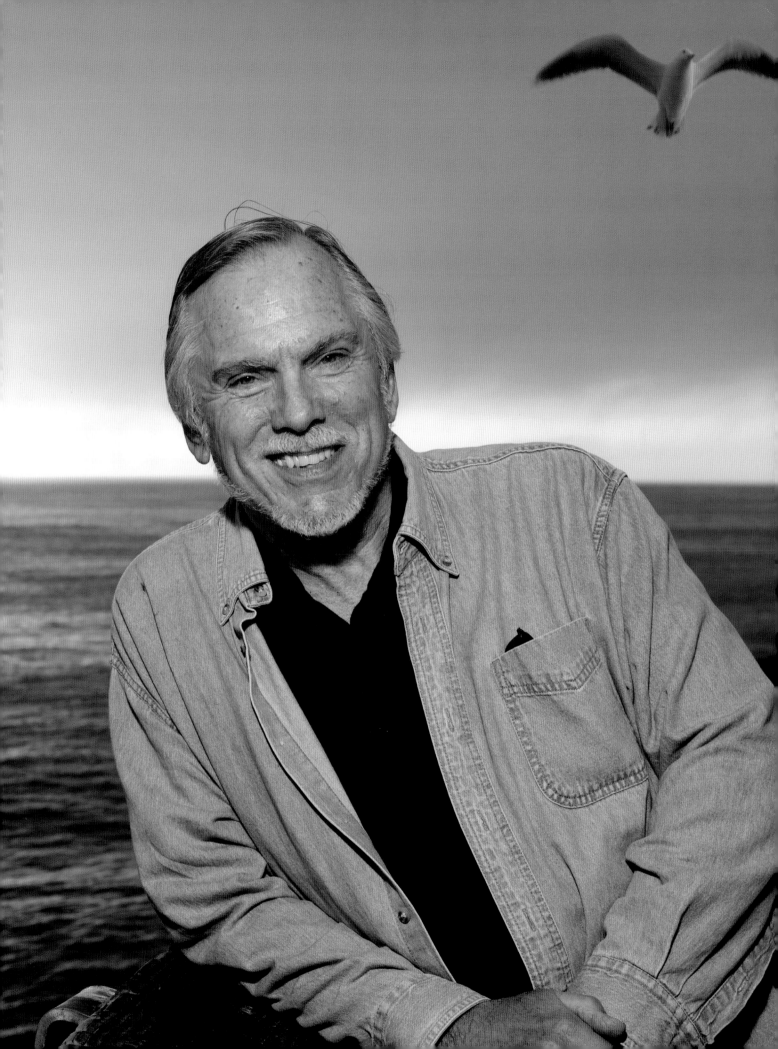

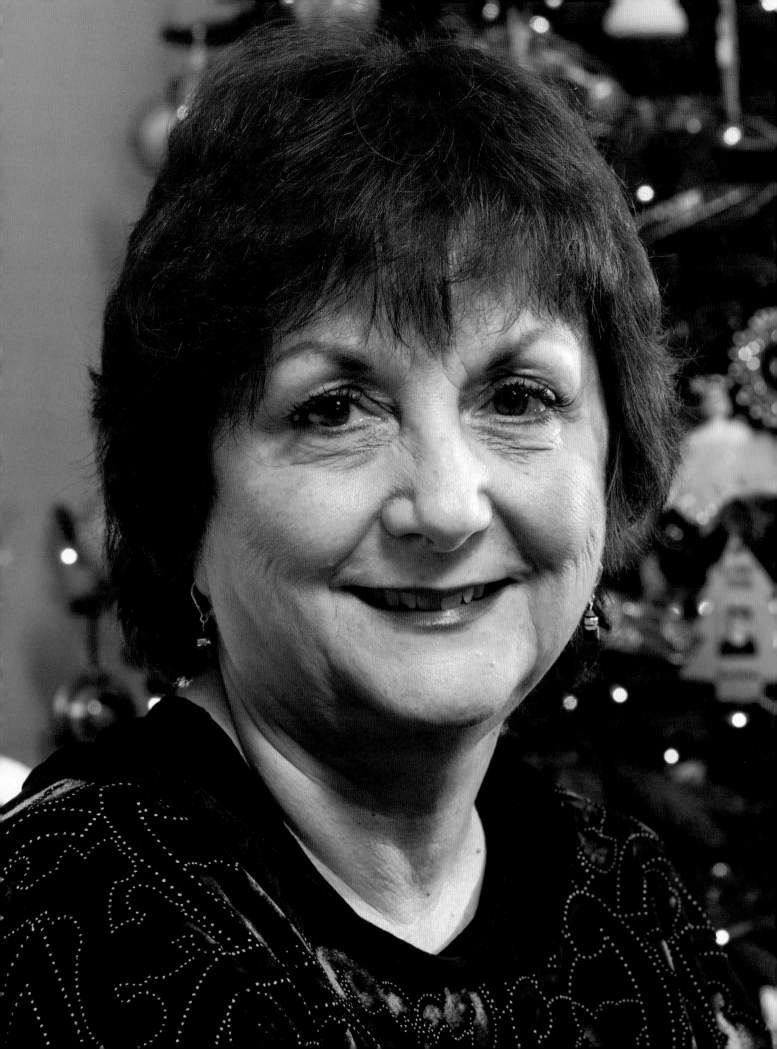

Cela Collins, mother of Dana Bell

Psychotherapist
Age at diagnosis, 56
Breast cancer, 2000
Recurrence, 2003

The Lakers won the championship on the day of my diagnosis, so at least one good thing happened that day. It turns out that a lot of good came from that day. I would never say that I wish it hadn't happened. I mean that honestly. It has been monumental to my life.

Having had cancer has also made me a better therapist. Any time you suffer, you develop a lot more empathy and understanding. I love what I do, helping others. My work, my family, and my life in general are all so full.

My experience with cancer has made me so grateful for all that I have. It also made me reevaluate my priorities. I love to travel, and thought of all the places that I had wanted to go to and kept putting off. Since then, I have traveled to seventeen different countries.

I have new priorities. I am now much more aware of my body. I used to take my health for granted, but now I eat well and work out several times a week. Spirituality has also deepened for me. I joined a much more liberal, socially-conscious church. It's very sustaining and so comforting to be around people who think like I do.

My daughter has suffered with the same cancer at such a young age. I don't know exactly how she feels, but I understand so much of it. We're sisters in our disease as well as mother and daughter.

Two years later, I felt something where my surgery had been. I had cancer again in the exact same spot, which is a very rare occurrence. Three days later, I found a third lump.

Beverlye Hyman Fead was awarded the National Profile of Courage Award from the National Sarcoma Society, 2009.

43

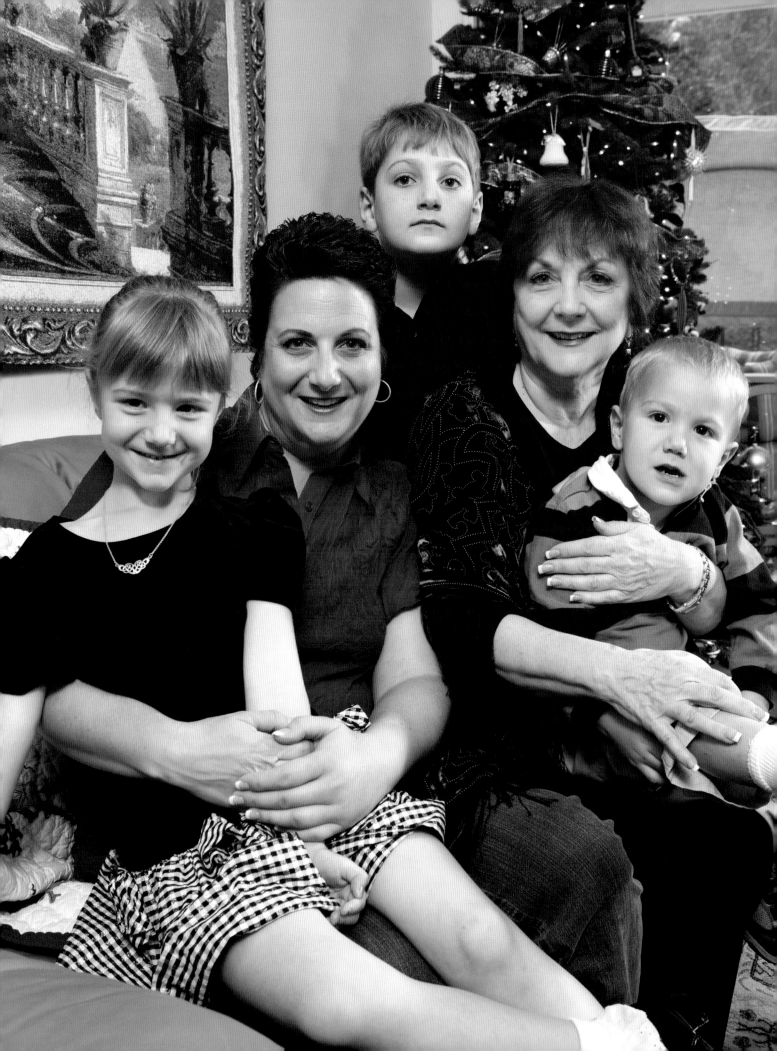

Dana Bell, daughter of Cela Collins

Writer, Mom
Age at diagnosis, 37
Metastatic breast cancer, 2007

*I*t was the worst year of my life. My son was diagnosed with autism, I got breast cancer, and my husband left us. I discovered the lump in my breast the week of Christmas, and had to struggle through the holidays with three children without their father for the first time.

My autistic son had a difficult time understanding. Instead of a lump on my breast, he told everyone, "Mommy swallowed a rock." And so I have written about *The Rock: The one that left, the one I had removed, and the one I have become.*

I had to become a rock, but it wasn't easy losing a part of who I am as a woman. You don't realize how much you value a breast until it's gone. Something that was a food source for my children, that sustained life, was now a threat to my own life.

After my surgery, forty girlfriends came over to the house for a head-shaving party. They each made a quilt square and sewed them together to make a quilt for me to use during my chemo treatments. I had gotten a whole bunch of wigs, so we decorated the Styrofoam heads and gave them names and personalities. After that, the kids picked one every day, and that's who I would become that day. I needed this to be a time to celebrate, laugh, and find strength.

> *After my surgery, forty girlfriends came over to the house for a head-shaving party.*

I'm moving on now and dating again. It's an interesting gauge of someone's sensitivity and depth when you tell them you had cancer. In general though, dates have not been turned off by it. I told this one guy that if the date didn't go well, I would change my wig, change my name, and show up the next week as a different date. I really never expected that anyone would be attracted to a young, single mother with cancer. It's been very validating and liberating.

I've made so many discoveries:

- If I can handle everything that happened that year, I can handle anything for the rest of my life.
- I need to be comfortable in not knowing what I don't know. I know nothing about my future. All I can control is my optimism.
- Now I know it's not things that make happiness; it's *people*. My life before this was "things." I have survived through kindness, not things. Sometimes groceries would magically appear on my porch with no note. Five friends walked in honor of me in the Revlon Run/Walk. I met them as they crossed the finish with my name on their backs.

The value of life doesn't get more beautiful than that.

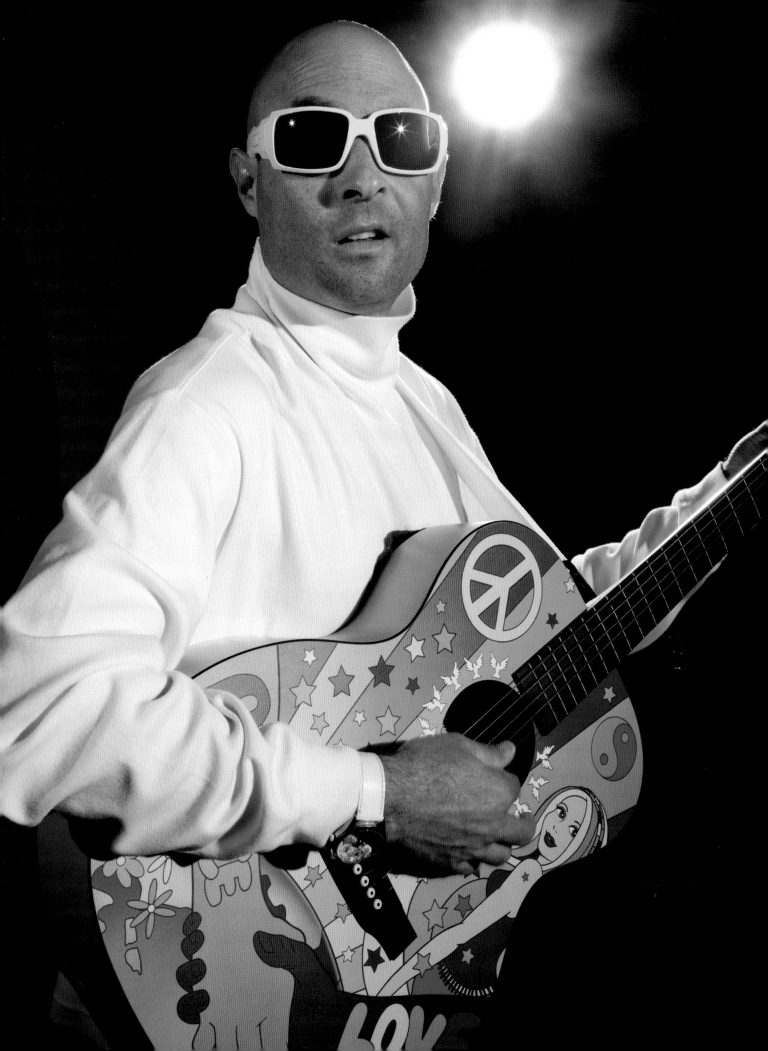

Charlie Lustman

Singer, Songwriter, Musician
Age at diagnosis, 40
Osteosarcoma of the jaw, 2006

I don't believe in statistics. If I did, you'd be listening to a ghost. A routine dentist visit revealed that I had an unusual lump on my upper jaw. The biopsy determined it was osteosarcoma, an extremely rare cancer. I plowed through a marathon, three-day vocal session to finish an album before going under the knife. Two surgeries later, I had lost three-quarters of my upper jaw.

I wrote a song for my daughter Gita, who was born on the third floor of the medical center while I was on the lower level receiving chemotherapy. When they handed her to me, I held her and said, "I'm going to be there for your wedding."

On the one-year anniversary of my diagnosis, I wrote a song about my experience with cancer. It is titled "The Call." The lyrics kept coming as I wrote about everything from diagnosis to surgery, from "chemo brain" to remission. It became a thirteen-song tribute album to my son Shaya.

> I don't believe in statistics. If I did, you'd be listening to a ghost.

Through my music I could process everything that had happened, and it also gave me confidence that I had a reason for staying on this planet. My newest album is *Made Me Nuclear*, which I have also turned into an operetta. I started performing my songs at cancer centers and then adapted the work for stage.

A friend told me not to let the doctors tell me when I was going to die. That was particularly profound for me because my father was a holocaust survivor. I never lost hope. I was determined not to let cancer be my reality. I want to take my musical campaign of hope, strength, and love all across America. I want to reach out to more people with a message of empowerment and overcoming difficult life challenges.

Chelsea Kauffman | Age at diagnosis, 15
Germ cell teratoma, 2005

CHELSEA: Before I was diagnosed with cancer, I was just another giddy fifteen-year-old, size-four girl. After six surgeries and six months of chemotherapy, I first had to learn that I needed to allow myself to grieve for all the fear that I experienced, and most important, the loss of my fifteenth year. Only after the grief could my focus change to moving forward.

I've been in remission for a few years now, and I've learned that pessimism is not the way to go through life. It merely kept me numb. It was time for me to start living my life.

I wasn't given my life back so that others could direct it. I got it back to celebrate it my way. I still haven't found out what that celebration looks like, but this is what I know: I love the ocean, Italian food, my family and friends, and my Jewish community. I know I want to be a doctor, and now I have inspiration. I can fight disease on behalf of others. I know I can plan ahead because my future now exists. I know not to sweat the small things but focus on the big. I long ago stopped wearing a wig and I have designed my wedding dress.

To live without goals is to exist without celebrating life.

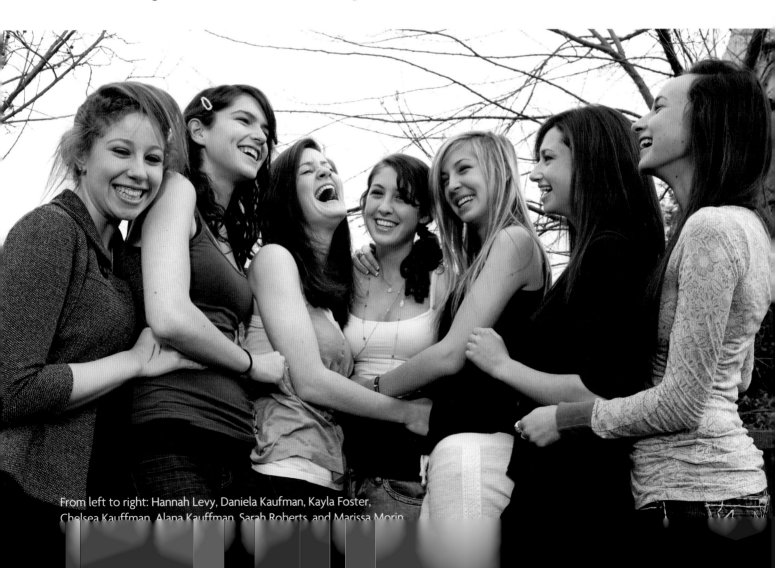

From left to right: Hannah Levy, Daniela Kaufman, Kayla Foster, Chelsea Kauffman, Alana Kauffman, Sarah Roberts, and Marissa Morin.

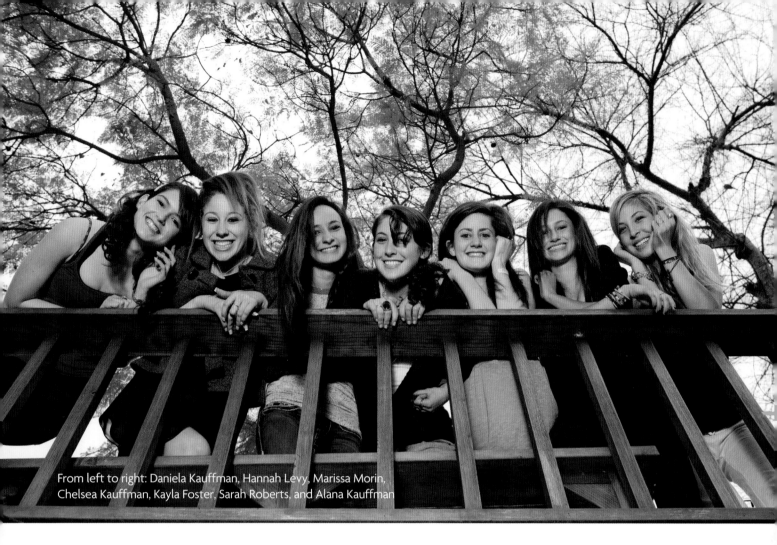

From left to right: Daniela Kauffman, Hannah Levy, Marissa Morin, Chelsea Kauffman, Kayla Foster, Sarah Roberts, and Alana Kauffman

To live without goals is to exist without celebrating life.

ALANA, CHELSEA'S TWIN SISTER: I have always been the nurturer and she has always been the fighter, so it was perfect how this worked out. If it would have been the opposite, I can't even imagine what would have happened. If I had to go through what Chelsea went through, they would have had to duct tape my mouth shut.

I didn't want to be the one to cut her hair, but our friend Hannah and I went and did it together. Afterward, I went home and called her on the phone. We didn't talk, we just cried together.

CHELSEA'S FRIENDS HANNAH, DANIELLA, MARISSA, KAYLA, AND SARAH: Of course all of this made Chelsea brave, but the weird thing is that it made all of us brave too. Two of us were there one day helping her throw up.

We would never ever have done that before. We would have died. But this was Chelsea and we just had to do it.

We were all so young and never thought about anything like this. So we took advantage of it and treasured our friendships. It brought us a lot closer, because we realized the importance of our time together. It was a reality check. Emotionally it was scary, but at the same time it was incredible how it made us all so much closer.

People can fight and get through it. No one deserves it, but she showed us how to be strong. Chelsea is our hero.

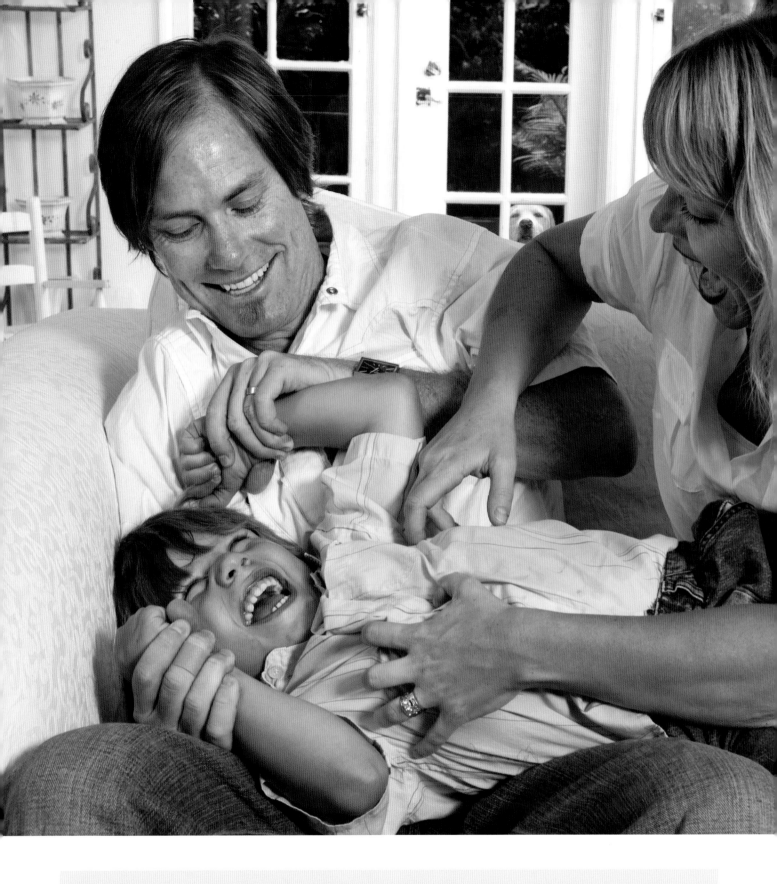

That's why I say, "Never give up hope." A door will open; you just have to make it open.

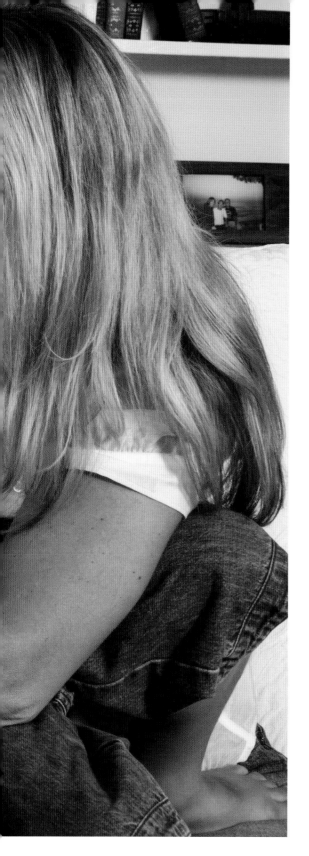

Christy Feuer

Public School Teacher
Age at diagnosis, 30
Breast cancer, 2000

CHRISTY: My first reaction was total shock. We had a plan, and this wasn't in it. We went from one day everything being fine to the next day wondering if I should have a double mastectomy. We were in the prime of our lives, just getting started, and this was a huge setback. We had to grow up very fast. We were young and playful and were going to conquer the world. Then cancer changed everything. It's supposed to only happen to older couples, when you're more mature and able to handle it.

CHRIS, CHRISTY'S HUSBAND: It's intense, particularly when you're young. But you can't let the negatives eat you up.

It brought us closer together. I believe the longer you're with someone, the stronger your love grows. The love settles in and becomes deeper. But as a caregiver, there are so many times when you feel helpless. That was difficult.

CHRISTY: Chris was right there with me through every step. He went to every treatment and doctors' appointments, and he didn't have to. I kept thinking, *Wow! He really meant those vows!*

All of our friends were having babies just when we found out that we couldn't. We felt so negative that we could not imagine something positive coming out of this. But there are no words to describe how much love we have for this little boy, Lucas, who we adopted. That's why I say, "Never give up hope." A door will open; you just have to make it open.

CHRIS: There's no guarantee that our own child would have been as awesome as Lucas. I would do this again if we had to.

CHRISTY: We have so much love for this little boy. I absolutely would do this all over again and not change anything, because that would mean not having Lucas. I wouldn't even think twice.

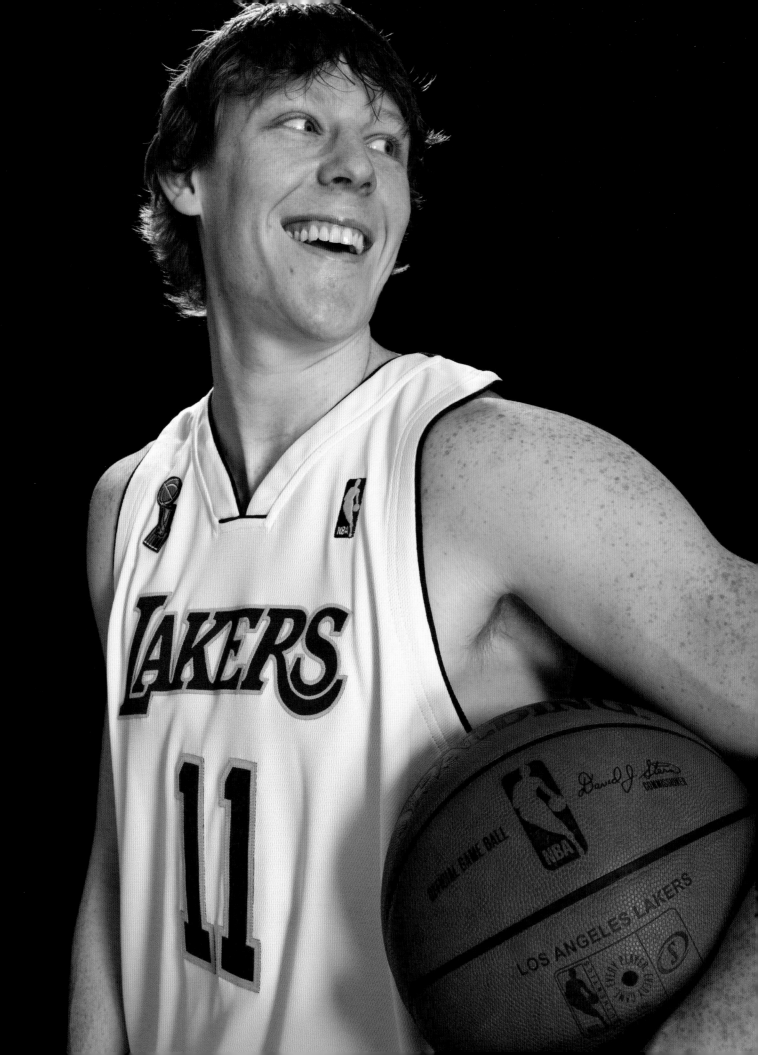

Coby Karl

Basketball Player, The Los Angeles Lakers
Age at diagnosis, 25
Thyroid cancer, 2005
Recurrence, 2006

During my junior year in college, everything was going well. At the beginning of the basketball season, I felt a lump on my throat. For a long time, they said it was nothing to worry about. Later though, my coach sent me to a specialist who did a needle biopsy and diagnosed it as thyroid cancer. I only shared the news with my coach and my dad and waited until the end of the season before having surgery.

In some ways, fighting the disease required the same skills I was trained for in basketball. I had to challenge myself to get through the situation, to focus. It's all mental. I am a competitive person, and this time I was competing against cancer. Now I know I will have to deal with it for the rest of my life.

Just six months after surgery, I was playing opening night for the Lakers, which was an even greater joy for me because of cancer. I know my dad is proud of me, but his is a tough love. The coach in him tells me to work hard every day, but, at the same time, his guidance has helped shine a new light on how to see my life and to know the things to enjoy.

My dad has always taught me to appreciate the little things. He taught me to enjoy my family and my team and all the great things I have, rather than looking at all the people who don't have cancer. You can't ask why. You just have to move on. If I keep that mindset rather than getting angry at the situation, life becomes so much easier.

> You can't ask why. You just have to move on.

Eventually, I want to be a coach and to have a family. It feels good to have a future to focus on and to see the possibilities ahead of me.

Conchita O'Kane

Jeweler, Painter, Writer
Age at diagnosis, 45
Breast cancer, 1995

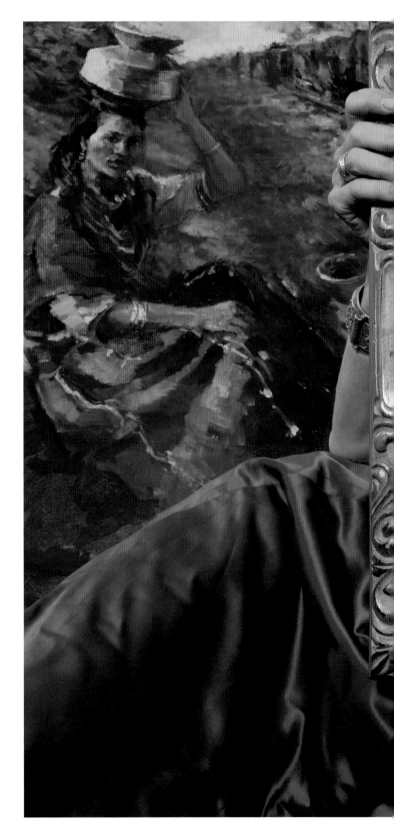

My mother died of ovarian cancer, my father died a year later of lung cancer, and then my sister got breast cancer. So, for me, it wasn't a matter of *if* I would get cancer but *when*. Doctors told me to stop worrying, but I still kept having mammograms.

One night I had a very frightening dream with men in burgundy masks, a bright green fluorescent ceiling above me, and a warm towel on my chest. A few days later, I got a phone call telling me that they wanted to schedule exploratory surgery because the mammogram showed a spot on my chest. During that surgery, the doctors were wearing burgundy masks, the nurses put a warm towel on my chest, and I looked up and saw bright green fluorescent lights above me. After that, I truly believed that angels could enter my spirit and give me a message.

Before my diagnosis, my relationship with my husband had been growing weak. We were empty nesters and going through trying times. After my diagnosis, he became the person I had fallen in love with. I saw his nurturing and his loving side. The relationship was wonderful again.

I began taking art classes. Creation is the opposite of cancer, and I developed a new passion, painting. I am in a consciousness that I didn't know existed.

I am faced with the reality that I am not destined to be around as long as I thought. It makes me push myself to more painting, more trips to see my grandchildren, more cards, more love, and more honesty. There is an urgency to reveal myself. I thank God for one more day. I was living before, but I wasn't living with passion. I will not be a passenger on the train. I want to drive the locomotive.

I will not be a passenger on the train. I want to drive the locomotive.

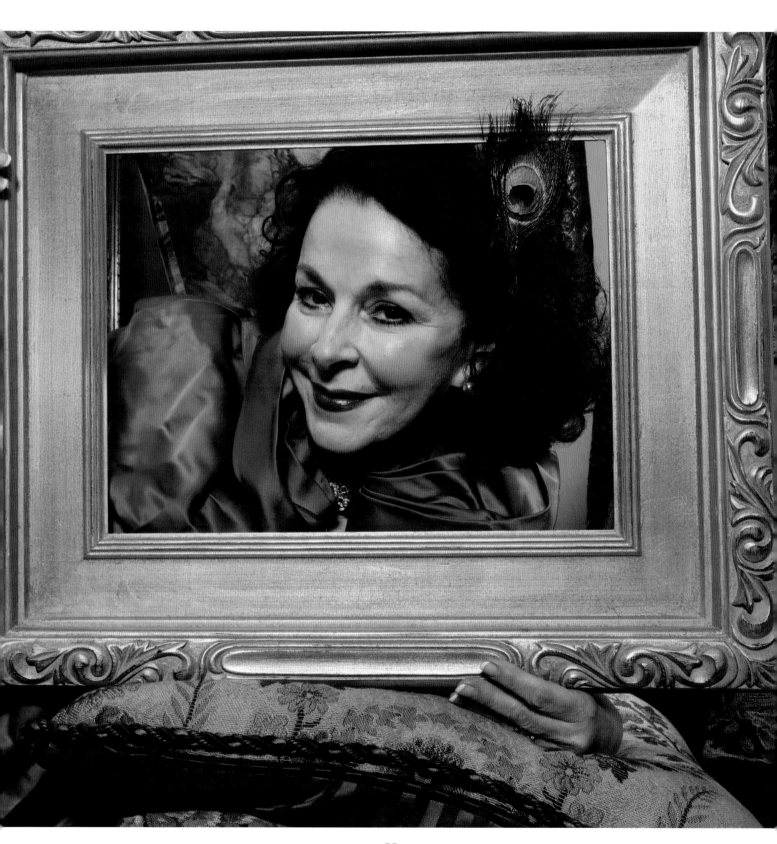

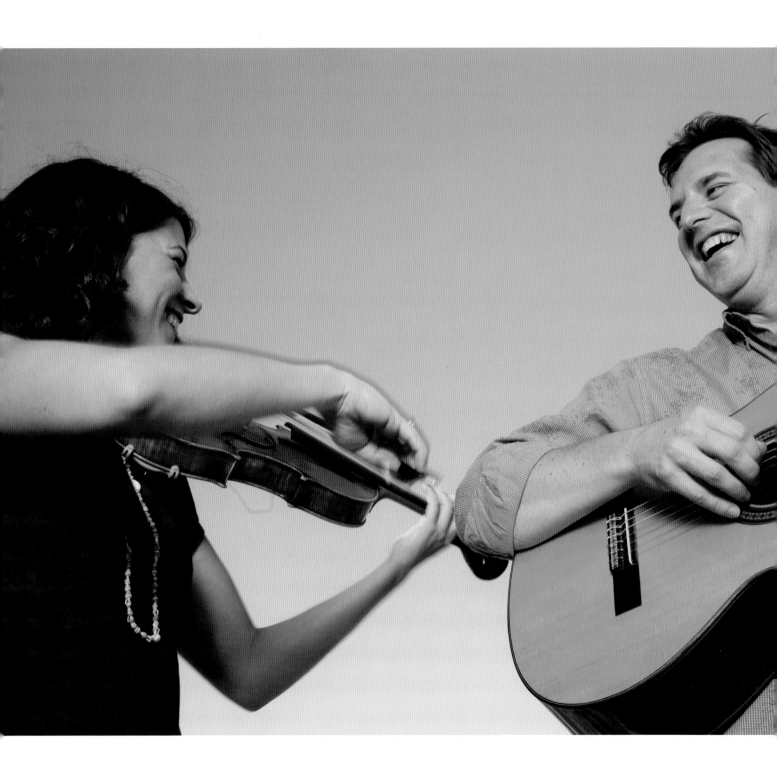

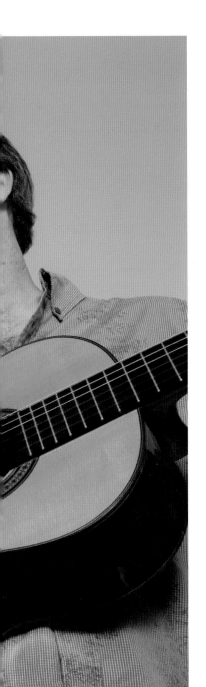

Corey Allen Jackson

Music Composer for Film, Television, and Video Games
Age at diagnosis, 35
Non-Hodgkin's lymphoma, stage 4, 2005
Recurrence, 2007

COREY: Immediately after they called and told me the diagnosis, I ran into the shower and tried to wash it away. I got out of the shower and smoked my last cigarette after a fifteen-year smoking habit. That week I went organic. If I'm going down, I thought, I'm not going down without a fight.

Cancer pulled my head right out of my ass. It made me wake up, because stage 4 is not just stage 4; there is no stage 5. As much pain as it's given me, the more I live with it, the more I get this overwhelming beneficial feeling. How can I not be grateful for that?

Like it or not, life is a terminal condition. And, without being present, it's over before the end. Work is no longer my top priority. There are more important things to do than what I was doing. Instead I am active in fund-raising and helping people. That has been very therapeutic for me. I also started karate again. We want to start a family, and I want to live to be eighty-seven. I am not so *me* and *work* centered.

SHARON, COREY'S WIFE: Every day he gets a cup of tea, and goes to sit on the beach. He doesn't work nearly as hard. Before this, the only breaks he would take were to get up and have a cigarette and make another pot of espresso.

Of course, it is difficult to see the person you love the most go through something like this. But I can say that my life right now is a happy life. That might surprise some people. We're much closer as a couple, having gone through this. We just celebrated our twenty-second wedding anniversary. He says he wants to live to be eighty-seven, but I'm hoping when he gets there, he'll reconsider that number.

Cancer pulled my head right out of my ass.

Courtney Dawn

Photographer
Age at diagnosis, 18
Osteosarcoma, 2005
Recurrence, 2009

After my cancer recurred, and spread in June 2009, I lost my leg. I am now four years in remission. But because I lost my leg, I have gotten crazy opportunities to be on TV, *Grey's Anatomy, The Mentalist*, and *NCIS*. It's been surreal.

I was diagnosed just after high school. I'm sure I would have stayed in the same area where all of my family lived, but cancer gave me a renewed sense of whom I was and whom I needed to be. I moved to Santa Barbara and attended Brooks Institute of Photography. My orientation before cancer was to barely do things. After cancer, I clearly felt like I needed to do more and explore more. It really opened my eyes and energized my whole life.

Cancer brought me to where I am. I'm more self-confident and I feel like I want to do as much as I can. I'm very happy now. I feel like my life is more fulfilled. I honestly wouldn't trade it.

It really opened my eyes and energized my whole life.

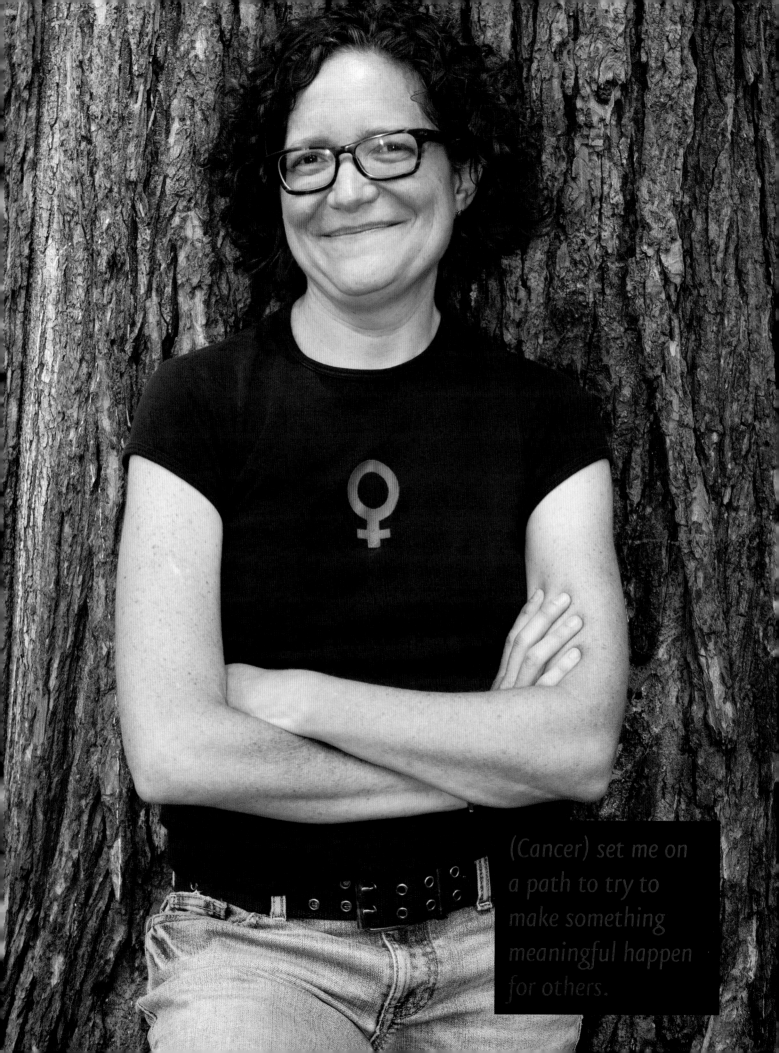

(Cancer) set me on a path to try to make something meaningful happen for others.

Cris Moldow

Social Worker/Acupuncturist, LGBT Cancer Social Services
Age at first diagnosis, 38
Breast cancer, 2003, 2007

I received my diagnosis in a phone call when I was at home alone. I was devastated. There's no way to describe how I felt other than complete shock. I never thought of myself as someone who would get breast cancer.

My father died of cancer when I was two months old, so I always had a voice in the back of my head saying cancer equals death. When I was diagnosed, even though I was told I had a good prognosis, thoughts of death filled my mind. I initially had a very hard time embracing the logical perspective that my diagnosis was one of the least fatal.

After my first diagnosis, I went through a single mastectomy and reconstruction, followed by eight rounds of chemotherapy. Technically, I was cancer-free. The second incident was not a recurrence or a metastasis, but a new primary diagnosis, also early stage, followed by a second mastectomy.

I was nineteen when I recognized I was not heterosexual. As a long-time "out" member of the LGBT community, I was troubled by the invisibility I faced navigating the medical system as a cancer patient. Because I was single when I was diagnosed, family and friends came with me to my appointments. While that was a blessing, I'm pretty sure I was not seen as a whole person with a gay identity of any sort, or with any human sexuality, but simply as a cancer patient. This was disconcerting, but more than anything, I wanted to recover from cancer, so I chose to ignore the issue.

Today I fully embrace my identification as a cancer survivor. I am privileged to have a strong support system. Friends, family, my cancer support group, and other resources were all there for me and still are.

At the time of my initial diagnosis, I was working as a social worker at an organization in Brooklyn that provided education and support for women entering or reentering the workforce. Soon after, I was laid off and decided just to dedicate myself to my studies (I was in acupuncture school) and to getting through cancer treatment. I could never have worked full time, been in school, and dealt with cancer, all at the same time.

After my treatment was over, while I was reevaluating my plans to change careers, I received a job offer running a cancer support and education program in the LGBT community. Accepting this job was a transformational decision for me because it empowered me to become a stronger LGBT and cancer activist as my own recovery journey proceeded.

Going through cancer led me to discover a much deeper sense of myself and set me on a path to try to make something meaningful happen for others. It's hard to know who I would be now if I hadn't gone through cancer. I would much prefer that nobody get cancer and that it be eradicated, along with countless other plagues we have yet to eliminate in our society. I think we're on the way but far from there. Despite that, I like my life now; if not for cancer, I know I wouldn't have this version of it or many of the incredible people I have met. There have also been silver linings both personally and professionally: I understand something much deeper about self-care, emotional, physical and spiritual; and I regularly work toward reducing cancer-care barriers and health disparities affecting a multitude of people with marginalized identities (pertaining to sexual orientation, gender, gender expression, race, education, language, etc.) in this great city (New York). Overall, I currently get to live a rich and satisfying life filled with potential, and for that I'm thankful.

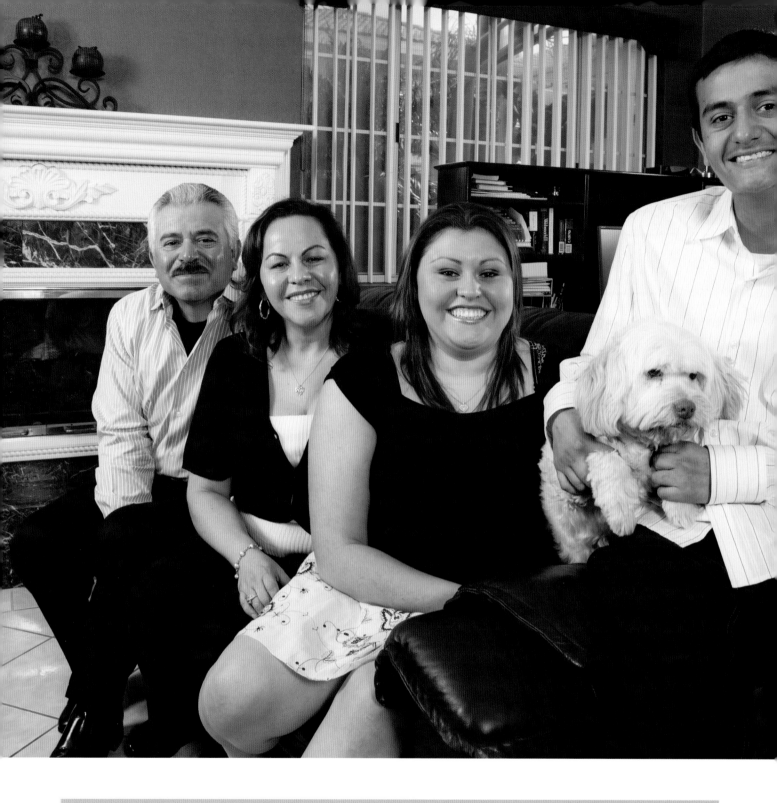

I'm strong because God is in my life constantly.

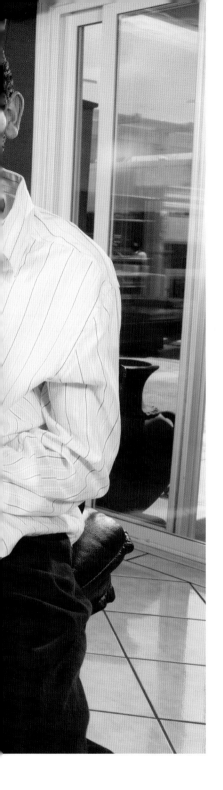

Daniel Lopez

Age at diagnosis, 17
Hodgkin's lymphoma, stage 4, 2008

*D*ORA, DANIEL'S MOTHER: Daniel has had numerous health problems his entire life. He was born with a metabolic disorder called Isovaleric Acidemia. His life has been nothing but doctors.

If I hadn't had cancer myself, I probably would not have been able to deal with his experience so well. We had to be strong together, as a family. We were forced to talk and share and be a lot closer.

We all paint this perfect picture of what we want for our family and ourselves. But as life progresses and we see all the tribulations and challenges that we're faced with, we think, *Oh, my life would be so much better if I didn't have all this.* But you know what? Not really. I see other people that don't have our problems and they're more bitter and more unhappy than we are.

> **The silver lining is God.**

When I look at Daniel and what he has gone through . . . so much pain . . . and yet he is such a happy person. He is blessed in so many ways. And he has a family that would do anything for him.

The silver lining is God. I'm not strong because of my own power or my own will. I'm strong because God is in my life constantly. I often say, "Here's another storm. Don't let go of me." He never said this was going to be a perfect world.

DANIEL: When I heard I had cancer, I said, "Is that it? That's all?"

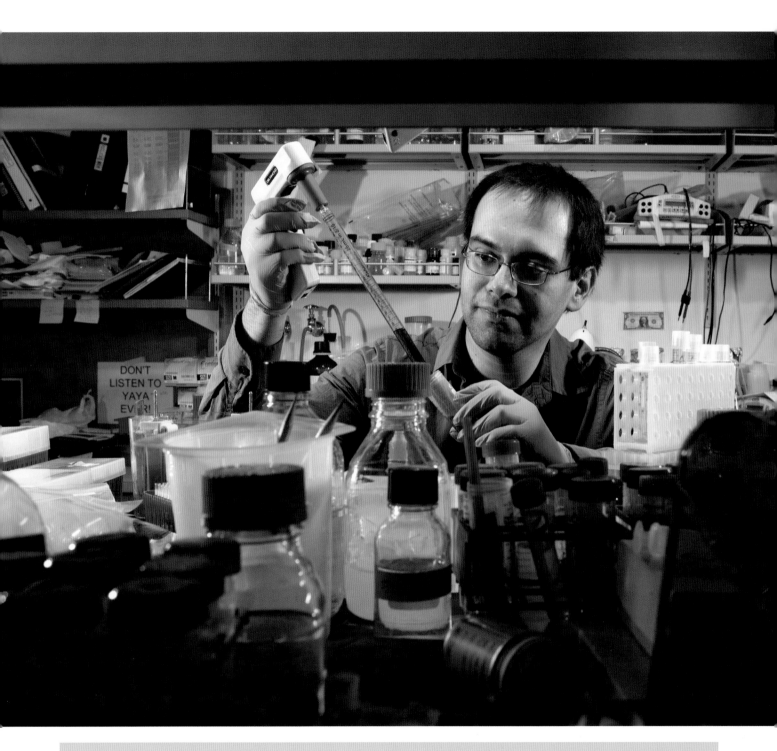

I use examples from my own life to show my students that the patients and cases they read about are real people who can overcome something as profound as cancer.

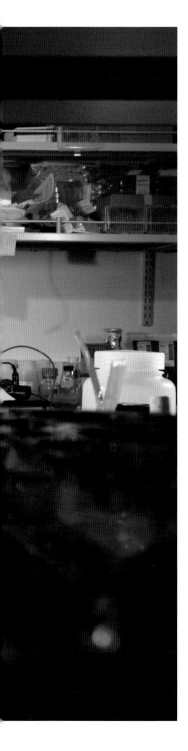

David Jesse Sanchez

Microbiological Research Scientist
Age at diagnosis, 19
Hodgkin's lymphoma, 1996

I was eighteen years old and just starting college. I had felt a lump during high school, but I couldn't imagine that I had cancer at that age, so I ignored it.

When I was in college, I discovered that the lump was cancer. I responded with almost no emotion about it until I had to tell my mom. She is a single mother, and I am her only child. My father died when I was two years old. I wanted to protect her, so I allowed myself to show very little emotion.

Since I was a biology student, I looked up cases of lymphoma, and, of course, the cases presented are always the worst ones. I went from showing no emotion to being freaked out.

My mother was able to take time off to come live with me at school, and so we had a chance to spend time together. Before that, she worked a lot.

My oncologist was like a grandfather to me. He was warm and personable to my mother and me. He also got me more interested in my biology major. Cancer made me curious about why disease happens. I eventually got my PhD, and I now study how the body fights off viruses.

At the end of my radiation, he told me to go out and be happy, and so I did. I said to myself, *I've already had that, so what's the worst that can happen now?* I took chances. I applied to good schools. I felt like I could do bigger things and take on bigger challenges. I'm not jumping off mountains, but I no longer worry that something will go wrong.

I had one long-term side effect from the radiation. It damaged my heart, and I had to have quadruple bypass surgery. I started to link myself back to the days of cancer, but I told myself to just get over this hurdle. The word is *fortitude*. It has changed my thinking from short-term to long-term. I might have to get through a few bumps, but in the end, everything will be all right.

Soon everything was back to normal. I'm happy. My mom is happy. I don't look back to the scary part of my past but look forward to my future.

I am now a professor and continue to direct research into how the body's immune system fights off infections. I also teach topics in biology to college and graduate students. I use examples from my own life to show my students that the patients and cases they read about are real people who can overcome something as profound as cancer.

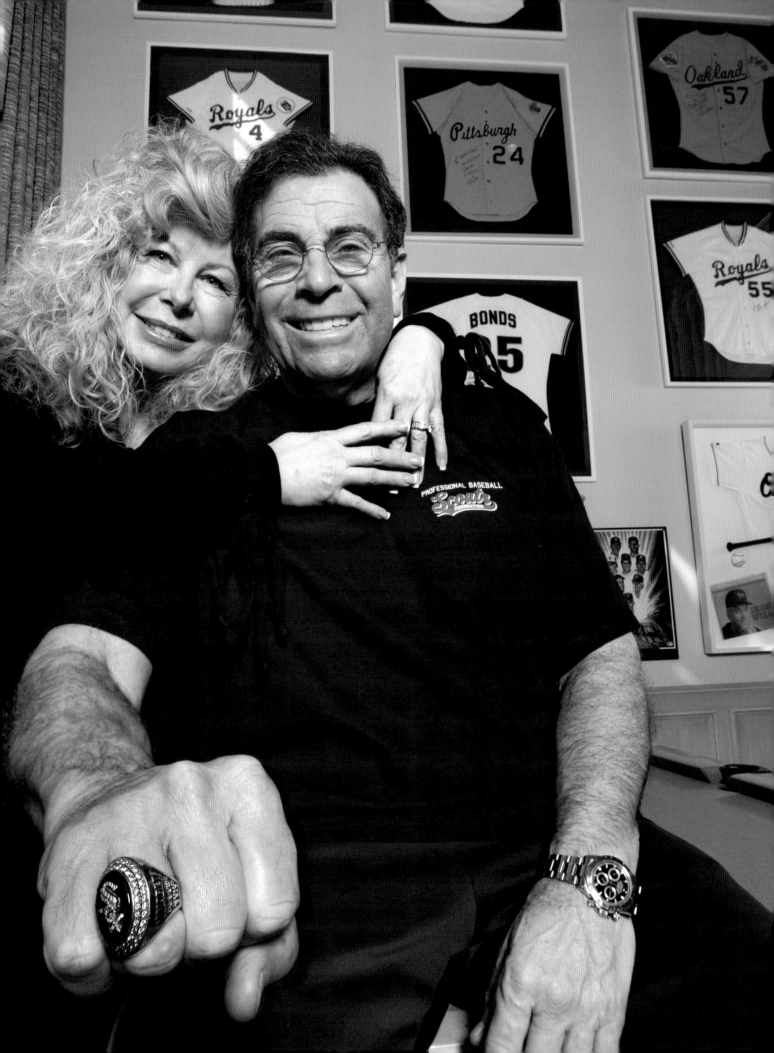

Dennis Gilbert

Baseball Executive, Former Sports Agent, Insurance Agent
Age at diagnosis, 56
Colon cancer, 2003

*D*ENNIS: My first reaction was shock. On my way home from hearing the news, I got a traffic ticket because I didn't stop at a stop sign. It was as if the police officer was talking to someone else. But once the news settled in, I just went on with my life. I went through surgery and a year of very difficult chemotherapy, and I still never missed a day of work.

My friends and my work saved me. It all had to do with my attitude. The medicine did what it needed to do, and I did what I needed to do, which was to not feel sorry for myself and to just keep charging ahead.

CINDI, DENNIS'S WIFE: I developed a sciatic back problem, almost needing surgery, but as soon as Dennis finished chemo, it went away. I realized that I had internalized my stress. Eventually, it all brings life a new meaning. I put everything in perspective and cherished the time I had with those I love. I've heard that so often, but never fully appreciated it until now.

DENNIS: Much of my life had prepared me for this. I grew up in an area where there were many ethnicities. I wasn't a big kid, but I picked up some pretty good habits, like fortitude. I had to work harder to eventually become a professional baseball player.

I almost look at cancer as just a hiccup in my life.

CINDI: He just always forges on, and I know that his positive attitude saved him. Diet and exercise are also two important keys. He has changed those habits a lot, but his work ethic will never change.

DENNIS: After my cancer, I funded a new baseball field in my old neighborhood in South Central Los Angeles. I also started a fund to assist professional baseball scouts, and we just had our seventh annual fund-raising dinner.

I almost look at cancer as just a hiccup in my life.

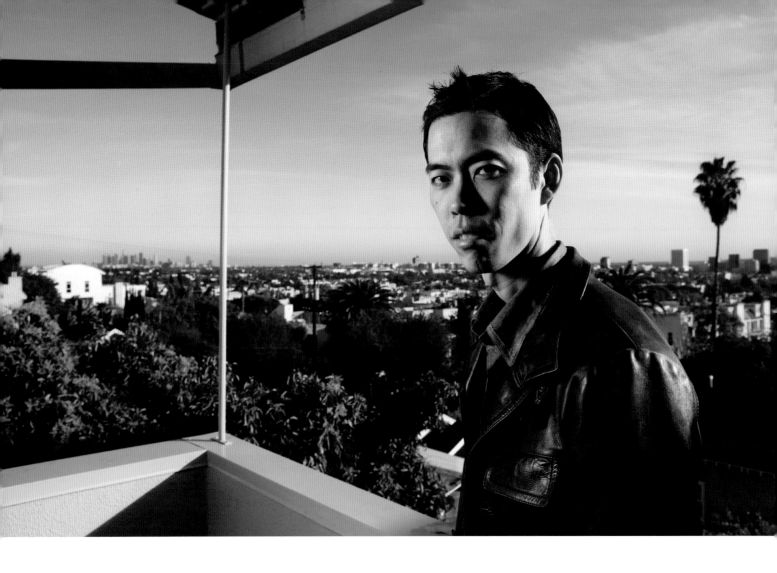

My grandfather told me that you will never look back at the things that happened to you. You will only look at how you responded.

Denny Tu

Executive Producer, Television Advertising
Age at diagnosis, 29
Nasopharyngeal carcinoma (NPC), 2006

*M*y grandfather told me that you will never look back at the things that happened to you. You will only look at how you responded.

When you're twenty-eight, cancer-free, driving around in a fast car, working really hard, and eating at nice places, there is no sense of time. You're forever young. When you get diagnosed, there is a change in awareness and a change in time.

When you are young, you expect life to come to you. But after cancer, you develop such a vibrancy and urgency to life. You have to go out and aggressively find the things that you love . . . if it is laughing, if it is eating, if it is cooking . . . you have to find what makes you feel alive.

Telling my parents I had cancer was harder than telling them I was gay. It was a hundred times worse. My mom took a lot of responsibility; she felt she must have given me the gene for cancer.

My career has done better because of the cancer. People feel that I am a little more human. They see me as a trooper; I'm vulnerable, but I'm willing to fight hard. In the business world, it seems to give you flavor again.

I think it is my job in life now to connect with people and to be at peace.

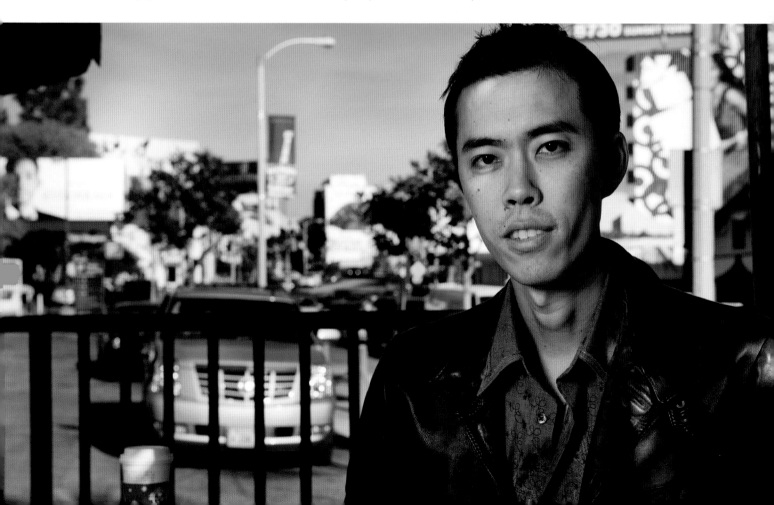

Diane Katz

Administrator at UCLA, Zen Practitioner
Age at diagnosis, 61
Uterine cancer, 2005

*I*t was the summer of my sixty-first birthday when I went to the doctor for my annual Pap test. After a follow-up appointment, I was told I had uterine cancer. Hearing the diagnosis was like being hit with a sledgehammer. I cried oceans of tears. A complete hysterectomy was apparently not enough; some lymph nodes of concern were found in the stomach area. And thus began My Year of Cancer, complete with chemotherapy and radiation treatments.

I knew I was a strong person. My mother had been diagnosed with breast cancer when she was thirty-nine and I was nine. And she went on to live for twenty more years, all before the era of chemo and radiation. I wasn't allowed to tell anyone because of the stigma of cancer in the 1950s. Many years later, my husband and I lost our only child in a plane crash. I had been through "tests" and had passed, and now God was handing me another one.

But there was something new in my life: a cushion, literally and figuratively. During the summer of my sixtieth birthday, I walked through the gates of the Zen Center of Los Angeles. I started Zen study, working with a teacher and attending retreats and services. When I began My Year of Cancer, I felt the support of my Zen cushion. I felt carried by the community of ZCLA (Zen Community of Los Angeles), sinking into its arms. When I was exhausted, they told me to rest; they insisted upon it. My teacher helped me to *be with* my cancer rather than fight it.

Before my hysterectomy, I had done a meditation on my uterus, thanked it for having served me well, and then said goodbye. My Zen practice helped me to manage gracefully through this very difficult period, to separate the facts of my life from my thoughts and emotions, and to see "just as is" without story and drama.

At the end of each week of practice at ZCLA, the chanter says, "When this day has passed, the days of our life are decreased by one." Those words taught me to take each day, each moment as precious, never to be relived or recovered, whether or not you have cancer.

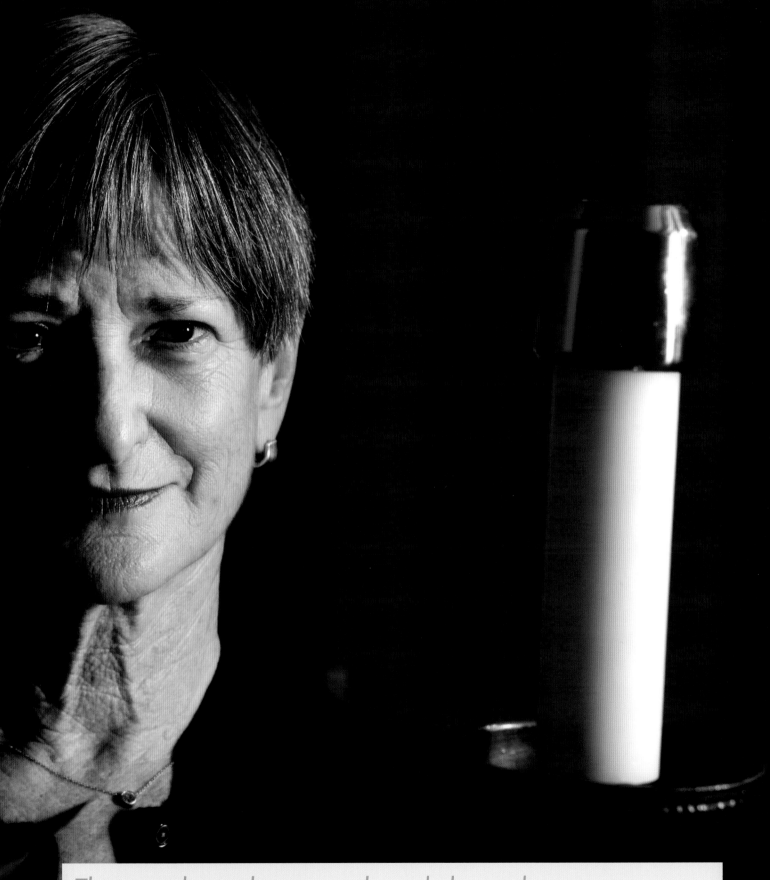

Those words taught me to take each day, each moment as precious, never to be relived or recovered, whether or not you have cancer.

Dolly Groves

Holocaust Survivor
Age at first diagnosis, 62
Hodgkin's lymphoma, 1998
Breast cancer, 1998
Cancer of the tongue, 2006

Amid the pain of the treatments for tongue cancer, I thought of my mother, trying to lead me to safety by escaping the Germans during World War II. Being Jewish, our chances were slim. After crossing into unoccupied France, we were caught by the Vichy authorities. Where had my mother found the courage to do what she did? She became my inspiration.

They call me the miracle patient. I have had three cancers, and this has changed my life entirely. I had to stop teaching immediately, and I organized my priorities. Things that had seemed important no longer were. I did a lot of things to make my life easier. For one, I don't argue much anymore. I completely simplified my life. I no longer cherish "things." We all go through transformations to teach us that things are not important. The only *thing* that I do care about now is my health.

I did something I always wanted to do. I started a company called Divine Design by Dolly. We make belly-dancing costumes. It literally saved my life. It's colorful, glittery, entertaining, and it makes people happy, which makes me happy.

*I did something
I always wanted to do.*

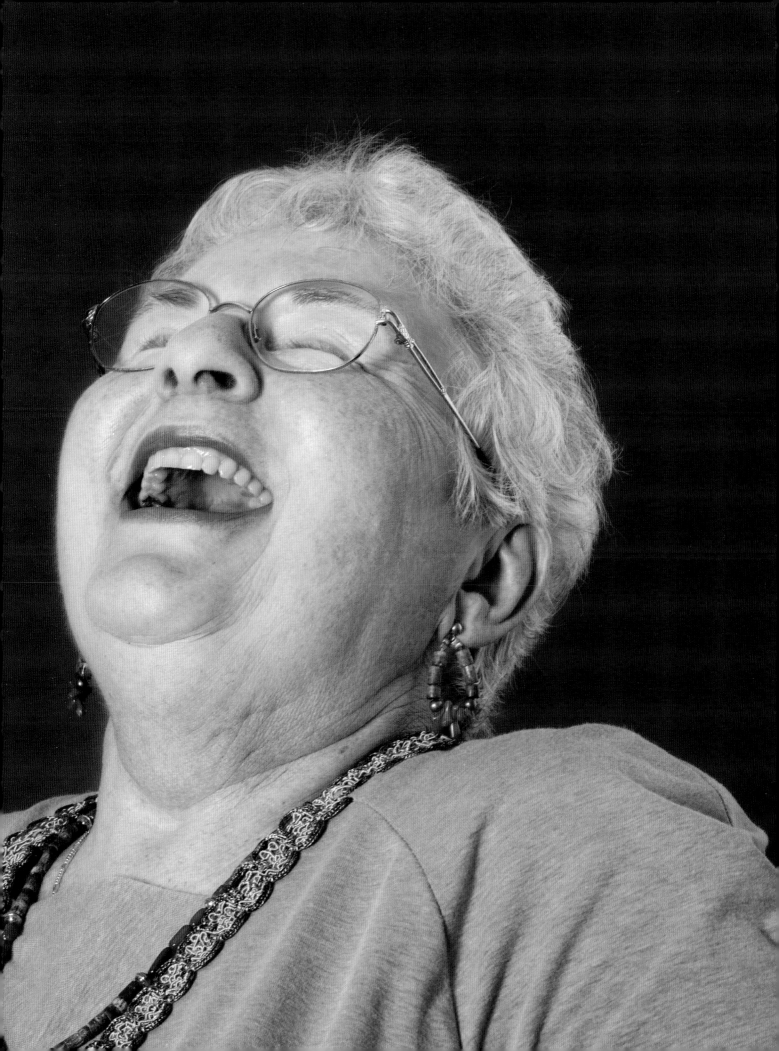

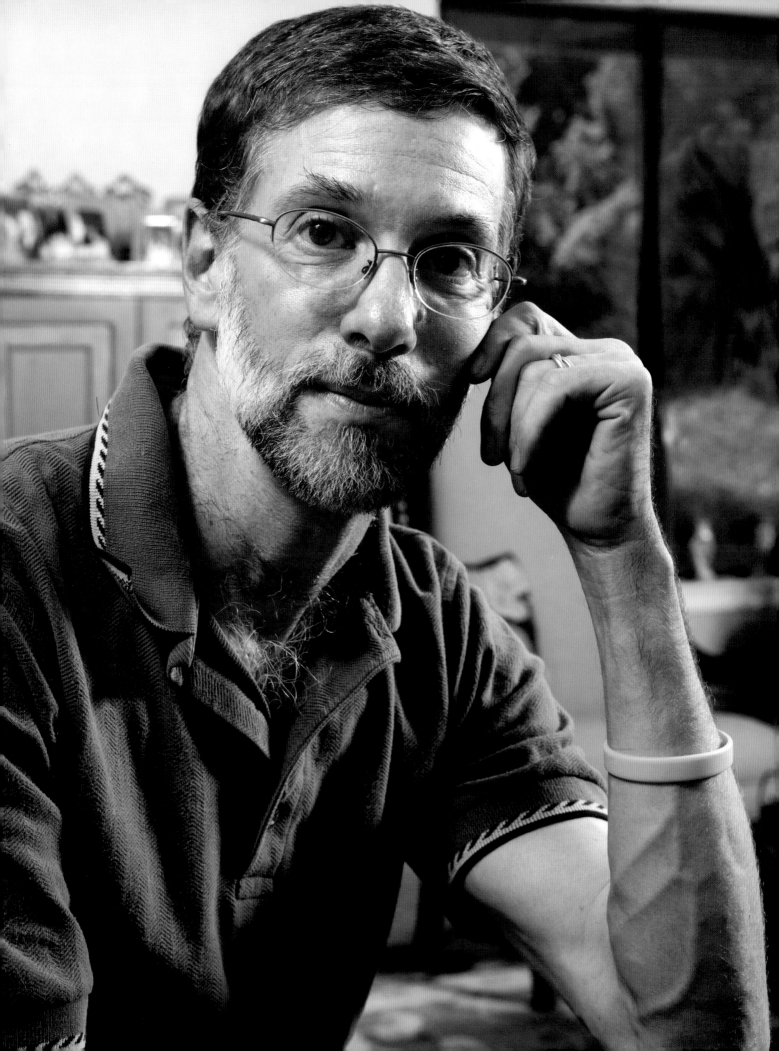

Doug Kohn

Author, Rabbi
Age at diagnosis, 45
Thyroid cancer, 2004

Since my diagnosis, I have learned from many cancer patients a counterintuitive truth. Again and again, they repeat, "We are the lucky ones." Lucky doesn't mean surviving. It means being who we are. And when we're able to own ourselves again, then the cancer doesn't own us any longer.

When Adam and Eve ate of the fruit in the Garden of Eden, their eyes were opened to their humanity and they discovered their nakedness. They were mortal. Cancer is like that fruit in the Garden. It opens our eyes. When we are told we have cancer, security vaporizes. Until that point, even if we're sixty, seventy, or eighty, we've got that sense somewhere of invincibility—that we still are able.

> *Cancer is like that fruit in the Garden. It opens our eyes.*

Cancer interrupts what we think is a standard trajectory of life. It puts us on a new trajectory. We have to adjust to the new normal. One cannot honestly have or face cancer without making deep and transforming discoveries. We are humbled. We are terrified. We love deeply, and we teach authentically.

What makes cancer unique among all other diseases is that it's a betrayal of our own flesh. My particular cancer has its own mystique. It's both acute and chronic at the same time. Going through the initial phase, it's acute, and for the rest of your life, it's chronic.

Since 2008 when my book *Life, Faith, and Cancer* was released, I have been busy speaking around the country on the subject of Jewish responses to illness. It has generated a new side of me—inspirational speaker—and it has challenged me to offer and receive responses in dialogues with the thousands of people I have met through sharing cancer. Who could have imagined? I guess we really are the lucky ones.

Doug Ulman

President/CEO, LIVESTRONG Foundation
Age at first diagnosis, 19
Chondrosarcoma, 1996
Melanoma, in situ, 1997
Invasive Melanoma, 1997

I was nineteen years old and out running one night in Maryland with my older brother. When we got home, I started wheezing. I had asthma as a kid, but never anything that bad. My parents took me to the emergency room, but the doctor said it was just an allergy.

Fortunately, my family physician happened to see the x-ray and thought it was a good idea to schedule a CAT scan. Soon after, I had surgery and they discovered a very rare cancer called chondrosarcoma.

Cancer changed everything in my life. There were two seminal moments because of it. First, after a long conversation with my parents, we agreed that I should go back to school right away to be with friends and my soccer teammates.

The other thing I did was meet with my soccer coach. He asked when I was going to start playing again. I told him it wasn't important any more, and he said, "No. When are you playing again?" He planned an

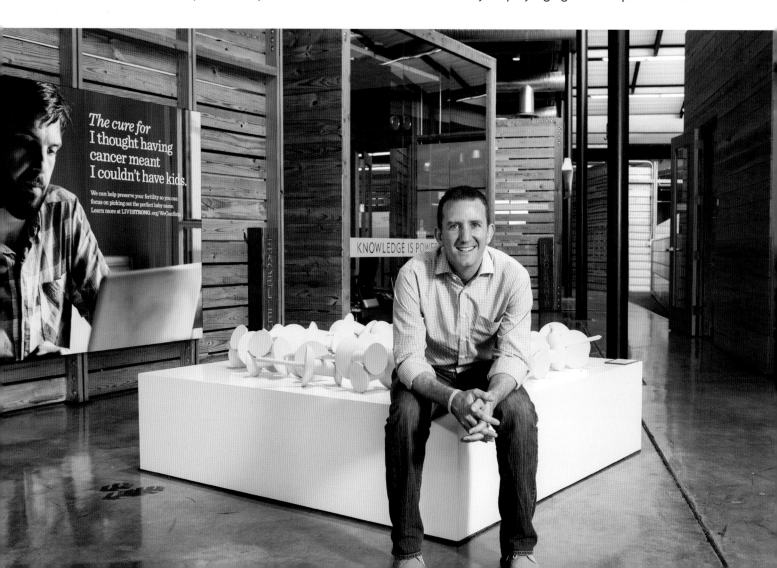

The cure for
I thought having
cancer meant
I couldn't have kids.

We can help preserve your fertility so you can focus on picking out the perfect baby name.
Learn more at LIVESTRONG.org/WeCanHelp

KNOWLEDGE IS POWER

exercise program for me, which taught me a huge lesson: You can set goals that might seem unachievable, but that is the way life is lived to the fullest.

I did everything he suggested and I was back in the game that fall. It was such a great learning experience. I could play soccer, or I could sit around and feel sorry for myself.

I could play soccer, or I could sit around and feel sorry for myself.

I also went on an unbelievable health kick. I was meditating, getting lots of sleep, staying away from cigarette smoke—all the things that other college kids couldn't understand.

I started a nonprofit in my dorm room to help other young adults who had cancer. I had no experience and no clue what I was going to do, but I knew there was a need and an opportunity to help others. Together with other volunteers, we created support groups, college scholarships, and a network for young people to become connected. The Ulman Cancer Fund for Young Adults is still operating. It has a staff of twelve people and it's one of the things I am most proud of in my life.

Soon after I started the fund, I was in my dorm room when my doctor called and said I had Melanoma. I had surgery and then followed the doctor's advice and started eating dark green and orange-colored foods.

The day I will never forget is June 2, 1997. I went to have stitches removed from the biopsy, and they found Melanoma inside my arm. I remember nothing else after the doctor said that sentence.

Since then, both of my parents have had cancer. Watching them go through it has been much harder than experiencing it myself. Being a caregiver is much more difficult. It gave me insight into how hard it must have been for them to watch their son go through something like this. My mother's dad died of cancer when she was nineteen, the same age that I was diagnosed.

During college, I received an email from Lance Armstrong saying that he read about our nonprofit. I met with the board of LIVE**STRONG**, and they hired me to help them build programs. Since that time I've been fortunate to work with a staff who has served more than 3 million people

Don't say no. Begin with YES, and have fun.

affected by cancer with practical, emotional, and psychosocial support services. We do this by creating a personal dialogue with cancer patients and survivors to inform all of our programming and advocating on their behalf for programs and services to their benefit. I'm very proud to say that we've been a leader in the movement to influence and shape the healthcare system to improve treatments and outcomes. It has been an unbelievable journey. We don't fight the disease. We help people. The disease happens to people, and we want to improve the quality of their lives.

Most people don't have a major life-changing event till later in life. I feel fortunate to have had cancer so young. It taught me to confront life in a completely different way. I used to be impatient about little things. Now I am impatient because there is so much I want to do. I always remember what my coach taught me; set goals that seem outlandish.

Don't say no. Begin with YES, and have fun.

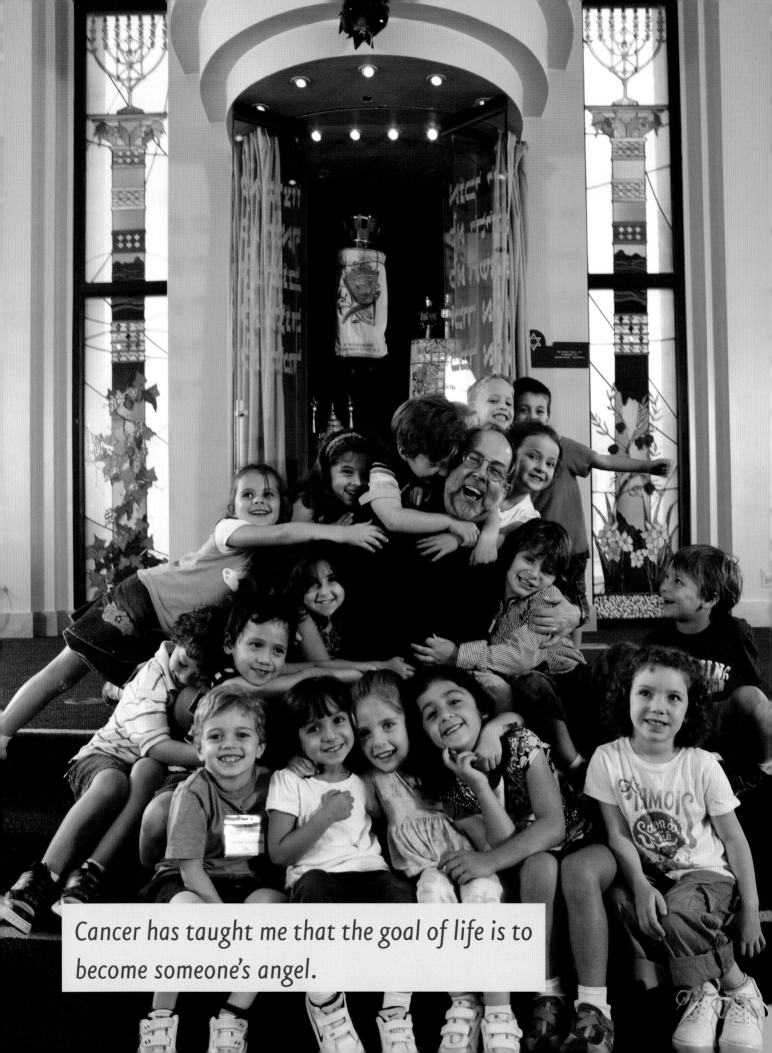

Cancer has taught me that the goal of life is to become someone's angel.

Ed Feinstein

Rabbi, Author
Age at first diagnosis, 39
Colon cancer, 1993
Liver metastasis, 1997

I was thirty-nine, a young rabbi and father of three small kids, when the first cancer was discovered. I had major surgery and a year of unpleasant chemotherapy. Four years went by and they discovered a tumor in my liver. The doctors were nice enough to let me know that metastasized colon cancer is fatal in about 80 percent of the cases.

It's chilling to hear the doctor tell you to go home and get your affairs in order. The hardest part was having my wife hear the news, and then telling my children and my parents. Once again, I had major surgery and another year of chemotherapy. But with great doctors, an amazingly caring and loving community, a lot of prayer and carrot juice, I've been healthy ever since.

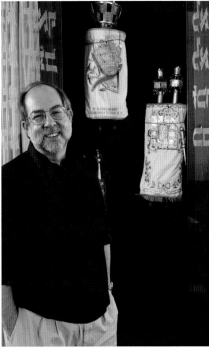

At first I had an overwhelming wave of self-pity, fear, pain, and sadness. I counted all the moments I would never see—my kids' bar and bat mitzvahs, their graduations, their weddings. Then suddenly I heard the words I had been teaching all of my life as a rabbi: I looked back at my life and counted all my blessings. I could have never dreamed that I would have the wife and children that I love so much. That I would work with my mentor and share his wisdom. That I would be surrounded by such a warm circle of friends. I desperately wanted to see my kids grow up, but I acknowledged how many miracles had already come my way.

The way of healing is to balance the loss and fear and rage with a sense of gratitude. When they balance, we are whole . . . whether or not we are cured.

I'm a rabbi and I have a pulpit. When I came back from the trauma of my cancer, I found a platform to share all my emotions. I realized that everyone sitting in front of me has his own life tragedies. Now I had the words for them. I had learned the way of healing. Having lived in the kingdom of cancer, I can speak about personal tragedy with an honesty and authority and humor that no outsider can speak.

I counsel people differently now. Death is not the universal enemy. Sometimes it comes as a friend and a loving companion. Some people need the courage to fight, while others may need the courage to accept. Everyone needs hugs. And everyone needs laughter.

I have come to believe in angels. In the most trying moments of life, angels appeared. Angels don't have wings or harps or halos. They don't float on clouds in gossamer robes. Angels are just ordinary people who do extraordinary acts of goodness and kindness and never ask anything in return. The world is filled with angels. It is only when we're most stressed, most troubled, most frightened that we see them. At those moments, their wisdom and guidance, their support and encouragement, their gentle touch make all the difference. Cancer has taught me that the goal of life is to become someone's angel.

Ed Schultz

Administrator, Radiology Department
Age at diagnosis, 39
Acoustic neuroma, Basal cell tumor, 1980

I was having hearing and balance problems, but the doctor kept telling me that I was young and just needed to get over it. They said it was all in my head, which turned out to be partially right. I had to threaten a lawsuit to get a CT scan. Then I had to get a court order just to see my X-rays. That saved my life. Eventually, at age thirty-nine I had surgery to remove my left ear.

Because of the hearing impairment, doing my job as a manager in retail was difficult. I sat down and wrote a list of my talents and my deficits, things I like and things I don't. I balanced that list with available

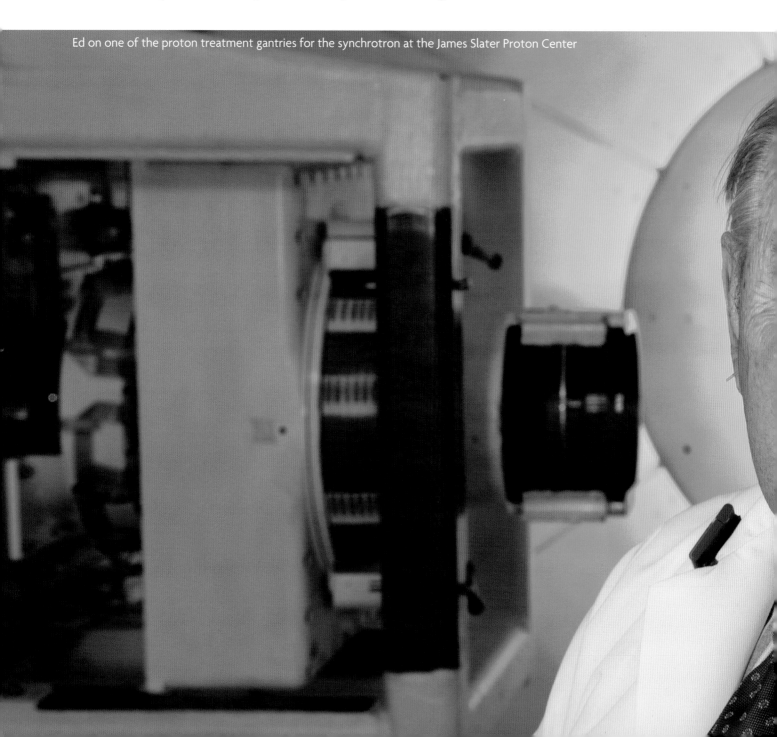

Ed on one of the proton treatment gantries for the synchrotron at the James Slater Proton Center

job positions and discovered that I fit perfectly as an X-ray technician. I applied to schools and was accept-ed with no waiting period.

I loved that profession, but I wanted to work with cancer patients to help them get through the process. Once again, a door opened. I was accepted to go back to school while working full time. Now, because of my own experience, I feel a kinship with these patients. You can't teach character and compassion in school. It is such a wonderful experience for me to be able to work with them. My reward is seeing these patients daily and making a difference in their lives.

My reward is seeing these patients daily and making a difference in their lives.

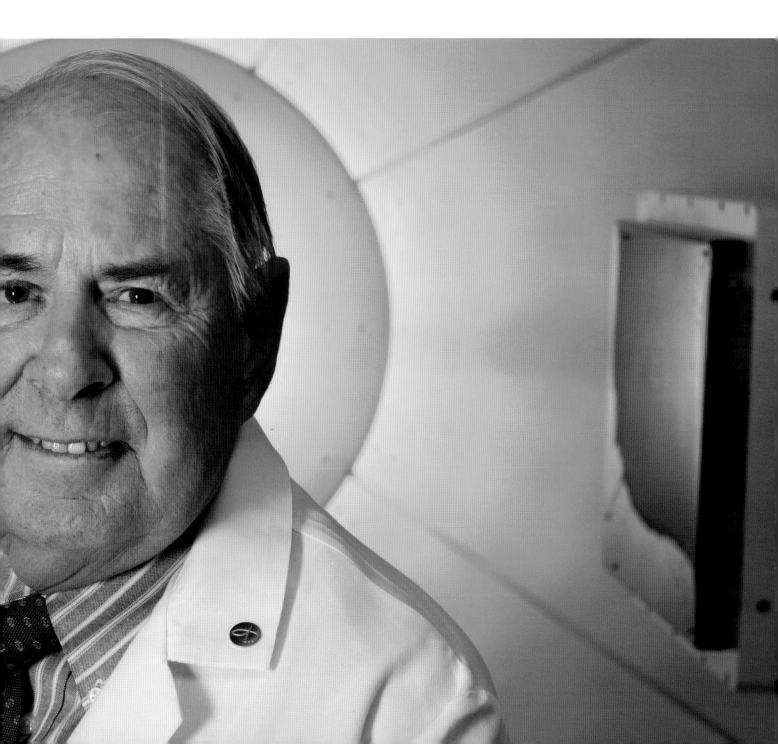

Ed Nugent

Software Consultant for Broadcast Industry
Age at diagnosis, 36
Brain cancer (Anaplastic astrocytoma), stage 3, 1993

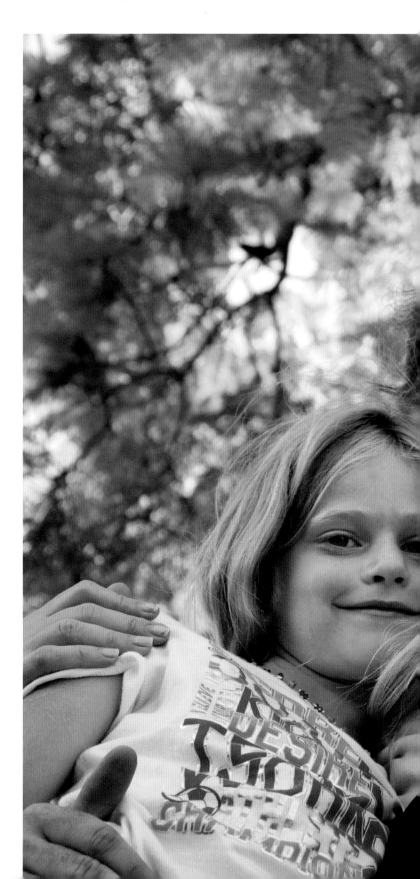

When I found out that I had a stage three brain tumor, it was surreal. My diagnosis was much worse than expected. I was engaged when it happened, and my fiancé had open-heart surgery at about the same time. So we call ourselves the Wizard of Oz couple; I got a new brain, she got a new heart, and we both got a lot of courage.

Before this happened, I was single, lived in an apartment, and basically just went to work every day. That was my life. Today I am sitting in front of this nice house, and I have three beautiful reasons for living . . . two of them are skating by right now. I wasn't supposed to live to see any of this.

I used to be hesitant about commitments. When you get your calendar put in front of you, you know it's time. My life became richer because I appreciate things so much more. My children can make me feel old, but I enjoy being a kid again with them.

I wasn't supposed to live
to see any of this.

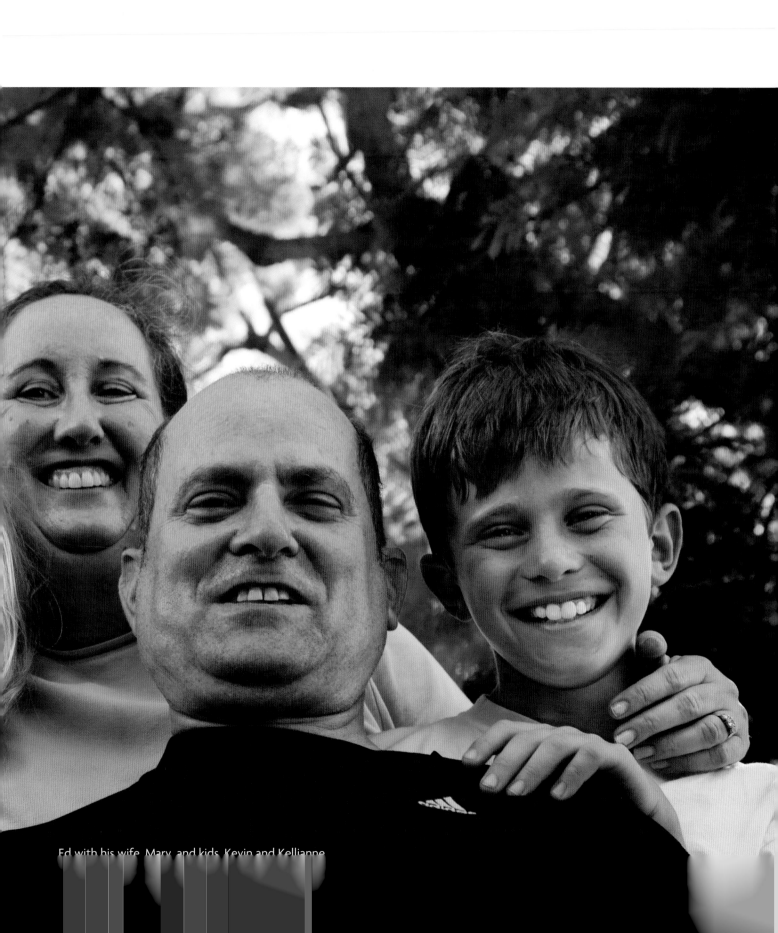

Ed with his wife, Mary, and kids, Kevin and Kellianne.

Elisa Hunziker

Chef
Age at first diagnosis, 45
Breast cancer, 1998
Recurrence, 2012

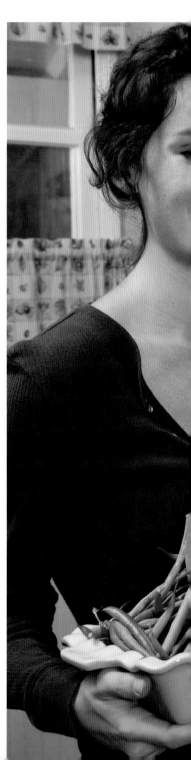

ELISA: When I was diagnosed, I was afraid of abandoning my daughters. Since I knew I had a good chance of surviving, I told them everything was going to be okay. I had a lumpectomy, but the margins were "dirty," so I had to have twelve weeks of radiation therapy every day. By the end of eight weeks, I was so tired that I just went to the doctor's office in my pajamas. One day as I was driving home, I stopped the car so that I could let out a primal scream.

LAUREN, ELISA'S OLDEST DAUGHTER: When she told us that she was going to be fine, I felt alright. Then one day I found her little leather journal where she had written letters to us in case she died. That's when it hit me, and it changed my life. It forced me to grow up. I started to consider life as more than just my daily routine. It separated me from my peers at the time, but it also gave me a new perspective. If she can get over that hurdle, then so can I if anything should happen. That's a very comforting thought.

ELISA: When I thought about the future, I became tremendously anxious. I decided that all I could focus on was today. I changed my diet to make "today" better. Before cancer, my family was eating whatever the grocery store offered. I got a nutritionist who shifted me to a nutrient-dense diet that excluded meat, dairy, sugar, and white flour. That transition was difficult; I cried a lot while cooking.

Because I was overly cautious about environmental factors, my kids have a running joke around the house that breathing, wearing clothes, or drinking water would give them cancer.

It wasn't long before I was enrolled in the Professional Culinary Program at the New School of Cooking. Now I speak, coach, and offer cooking lessons to help others learn the healing power of nutrition (cancersurvivorchef.com). It has been very gratifying to cook for so many interesting and lovely people working to survive their cancer.

EMILY, ELISA'S YOUNGEST DAUGHTER: Mom thinks she's hiding the flax seeds in my peanut butter and jelly sandwiches, but I know they're there, and I know she puts them there with love.

ELISA: I had a dream one night soon after I finished treatment the first time. I was young and I was standing outside my mother's bedroom door. She came out of her bedroom in her nightgown and put her arm around me and told me I was going to be fine. It was a love I had never felt from her. After that dream, I knew I was going to be fine. It renewed my faith in love.

Mom thinks she's hiding the flax seeds in my peanut butter and jelly sandwiches, but I know they're there, and I know she puts them there with love.

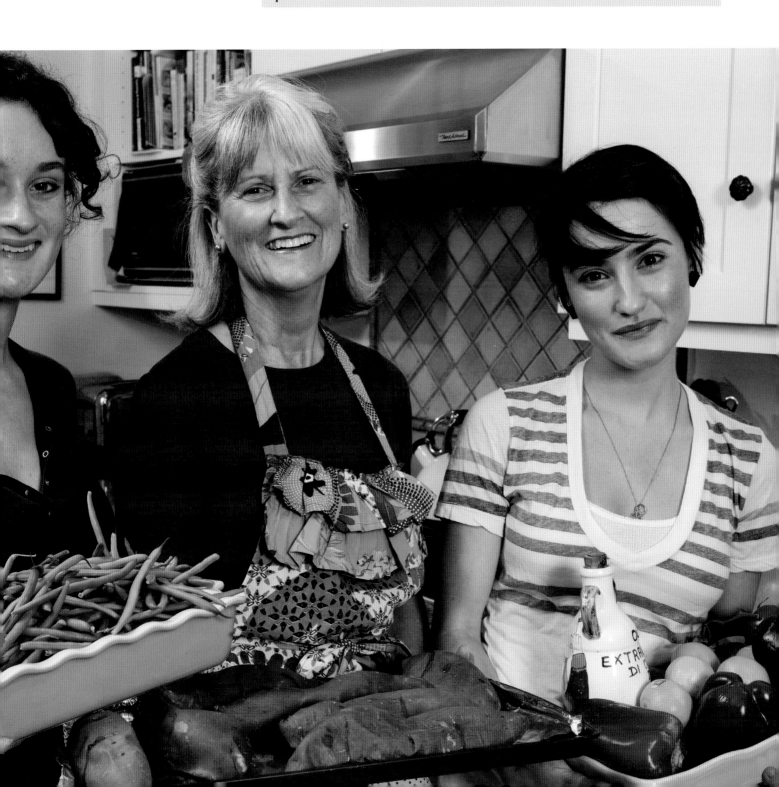

I'm much more apt to try new things. If I fail, then big deal.

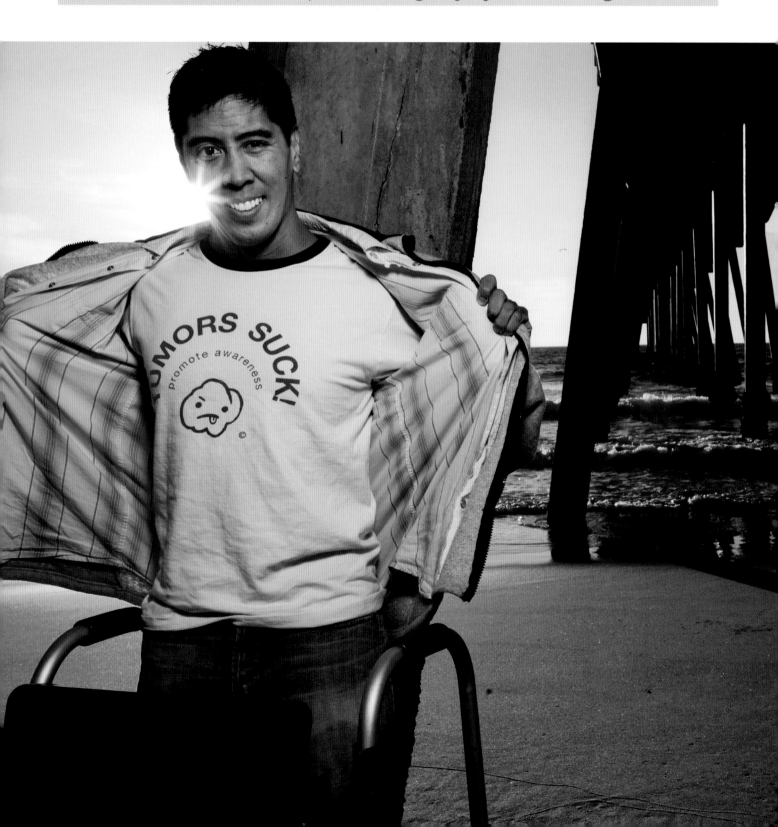

Eric Anthony Galvez

Writer, Philanthropist, Creator of "mAssKickers.com" and "TumorsSuck.com," Self-Proclaimed Professional Goofball
Age at diagnosis, 30
Brain tumor, 2005

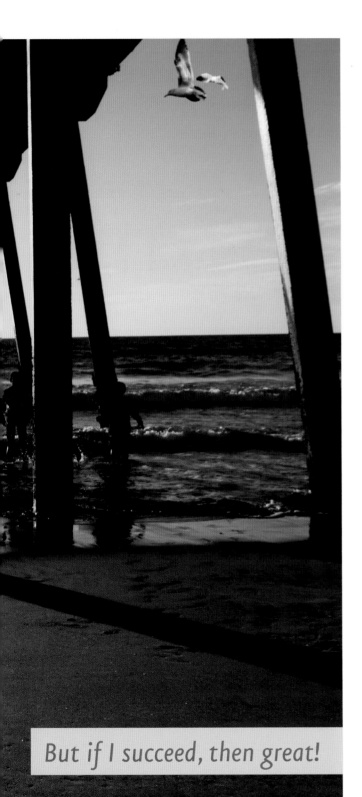

But if I succeed, then great!

Because of side effects from my brain surgery, I've had to relearn balance and coordination. I've done some 5K charity walks, and I'm trying to start surfing again. Before the surgery, I was doing triathlons and marathons. Having a walker now is a big adjustment for me. My improvements are what keep me going.

I know that being physically active before this helped prepare me for my healing. I have a doctorate in physical therapy (DPT), so I have a unique perspective on all of this. Plus, I've always been stubborn and a bit of a smart ass. Everything worked together.

It's convenient being a physical therapist, because when my insurance ran out, I started treating myself.

I woke up one day and said, "This really sucks. I don't want anyone else to have to go through this." I wanted to make sure that other people aren't as scared as I was, so I started writing. Typing was a bit difficult because I have ataxia in my left hand and a tremor in my right hand. An article I wrote for the National Brain Tumor Society turned into a book, *Reversal: When a Therapist Becomes a Patient*.

I really want to empower newly diagnosed patients. I have recently finished my second book, and the nonprofit organization that I started, "mAss Kickers Foundation," is now international. Last year, we went overseas to Hawaii, Japan, and the Philippines, with more to come.

I surprised myself that I've been able to get organized and pull all this off. I'm definitely more creative now. Before this I was always a go-with-the-flow kind of guy. I also never liked being in the spotlight. Now, everything I'm pursuing is putting me there. I'm much more apt to try new things. If I fail, then big deal. That just means I learned something. But if I succeed, then great!

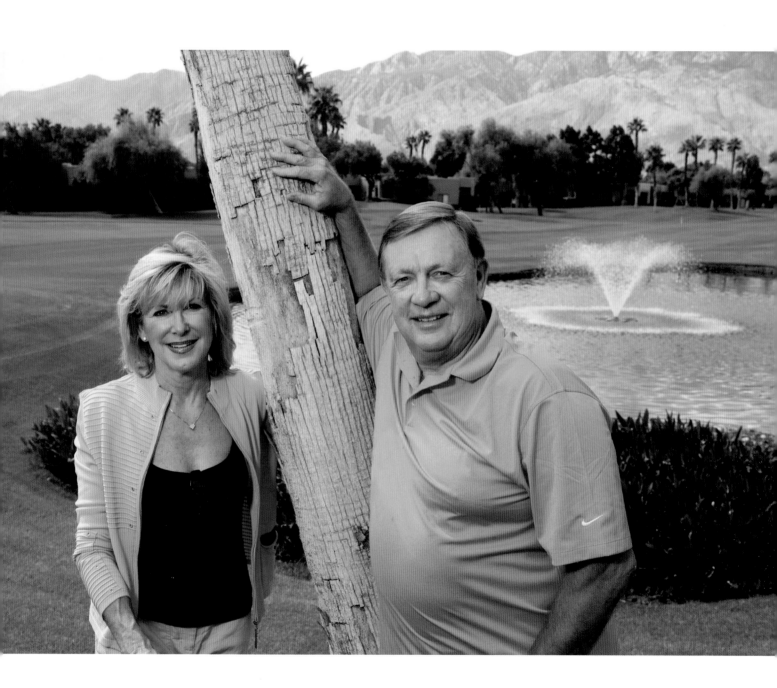

Gary Culpepper

Commercial Contractor, Developer
Age at diagnosis, 58
Prostate cancer, 2003

It took thirty biopsies to finally find cancer. We then interviewed fourteen doctors and I talked to more than seventy prostate cancer patients. I compiled three notebooks of information.

I chose proton radiation therapy and joined a support group of other patients going through the same treatment. The group was one of the most fun times of my life. There was laughter, camaraderie, and a positive attitude. You wouldn't know you were sitting in a room full of people going through cancer treatment because we all laughed so hard.

Growing up, I thought cancer was the kiss of death. Now I recognize how many survivors there are.

I was treated physically, mentally, emotionally, and spiritually. Because of Alcoholics Anonymous, I felt like my life was a miracle before cancer. After AA, I started listening to Him. God directed me. I talk to Him all the time. He speaks through my heart. My heart is my telephone to God.

Cancer was just another peg in my life. Sobriety was the key. If I hadn't gotten sober, I would have just let cancer kill me.

Now I have a job to do, to spread the word. It's what I was placed on earth to do.

Growing up, I thought cancer was the kiss of death.
Now I recognize how many survivors there are.

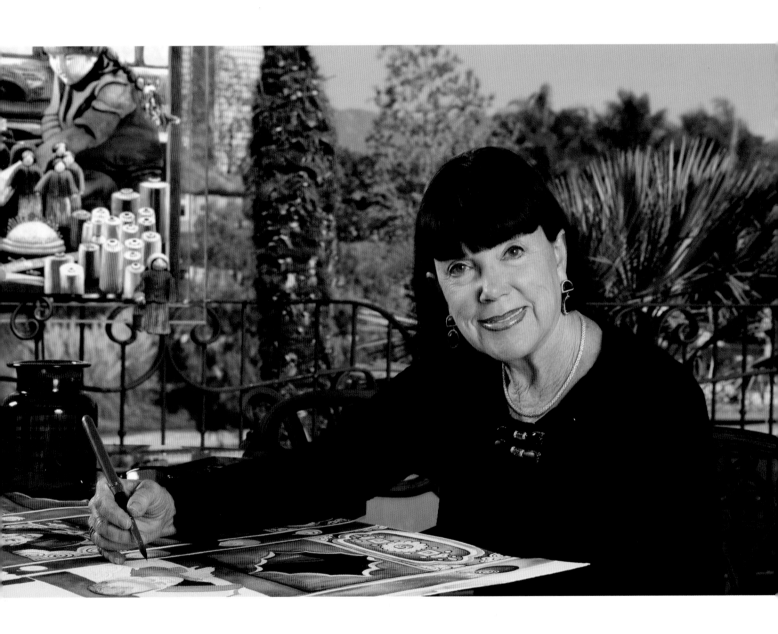

Gayle Garner Roskies

Artist
Age at diagnosis, 42
Uterine cancer, 1993

I was determined to be in charge of my own health. I was going through some difficult challenges in my life and in my mind, so it was no accident that I got cancer. I had been putting energies on things I could not control. I was having problems with my son, and the cancer was in my uterus. That was no coincidence either.

When they told me that they wanted me to go through radiation, I had a very difficult time understanding the rationale of tearing down your body so you can build it up. My husband could not believe that I wouldn't listen to the doctors, and my children were angry, but I made my decision. I'm very resourceful, so I looked into everything. When I went to the doctor every few months, he would write down what I was doing and just shake his head.

I don't know what really cured me. One thing that helped me as an artist was to draw my cancer. I kept a journal with drawings of the cells and my army that was fighting them. At first, the art was red and angry. Now I paint in bright colors and live my life that way too.

> *I changed "cancer" to "can survive."*

I also learned that I had to change the word *cancer*. It is the most unmentionable word I can imagine, even more than any swear word. No one wants to use that word because it means death. So I changed "cancer" to "can survive."

I was evolving personally at the same time I was battling cancer. I had always been a daughter or a wife; for the first time, I wanted to be me. My cancer became empowering. It was the biggest thing that ever happened to me. It was the beginning of me taking charge. I changed from doing what I thought others wanted me to do, to doing what I really wanted to do.

Cancer brought me to the fact that I may not be here very long. When I was fifty I ran the Los Angeles Marathon and I climbed Kilimanjaro. Those had never been goals of mine before cancer. But I did it, and I learned about my own power. Once you determine your own strength, then you can redirect it into all areas of your life. Cancer helped me take control of my entire life.

Because of how I changed, whenever I sign my name now, I write "Bright colors and best wishes." Always live your life in bright colors.

> *. . . whenever I sign my name now, I write "Bright colors and best wishes."*

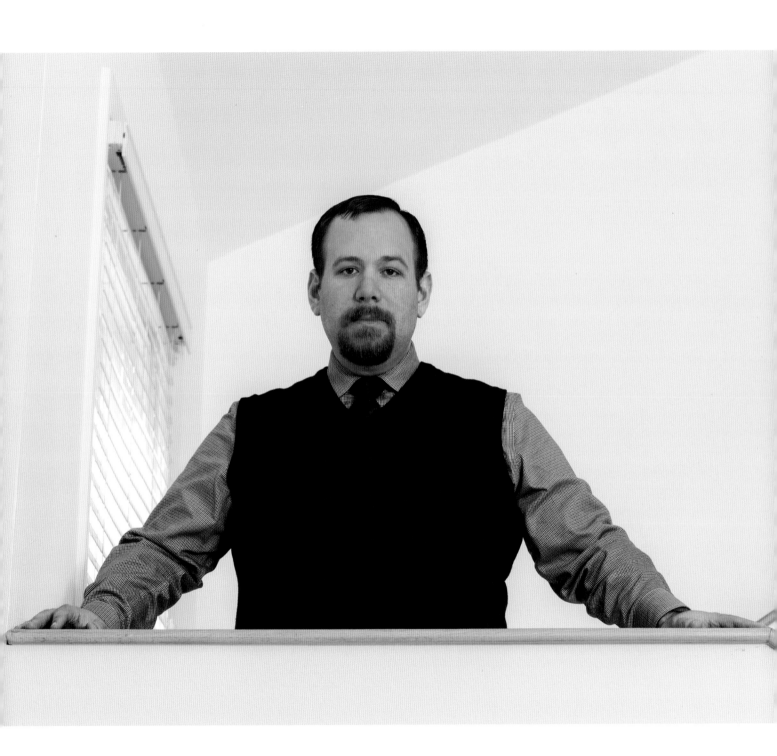

Graham Lubinsky

Physician
Age at diagnosis, 15
Pilocytic astrocytoma, 1997

I had surgery for a brain tumor when I was fifteen. A few years later, when I was a junior in college in May of 2003, I had a seizure as a result of an injury from the surgery. My IQ is in the 99th percentile, but my processing speed and reading speed were at a seventh grade level. I had to relearn how to learn.

I was used to doing everything myself, not needing anyone's help. When I started having these problems, I didn't want to face what was happening. It wasn't until I started accepting help that everything started to change.

Young adults and teenagers are already dealing with change. Cancer is like throwing a wrench in the works, and young people are often not equipped to cope. And yet, cancer has allowed me to appreciate life more. Before, I was just going through the motions. I didn't appreciate what I had until it was taken away from me.

My cancer, its treatment, and its aftermath have caused a five-year lag in my education. Nonetheless, I have since graduated from Michigan State University College of Human Medicine, where I served as the student council

I would not, however, trade the experiences of those "missing" five years for anything.

president and established a peer-mentoring program. After graduation in 2013, I moved to Washington, DC, and I am currently two months into my anesthesiology residency.

I would not, however, trade the experiences of those "missing" five years for anything. The struggles I've gone through will make me a more compassionate and well-rounded physician and human being.

93

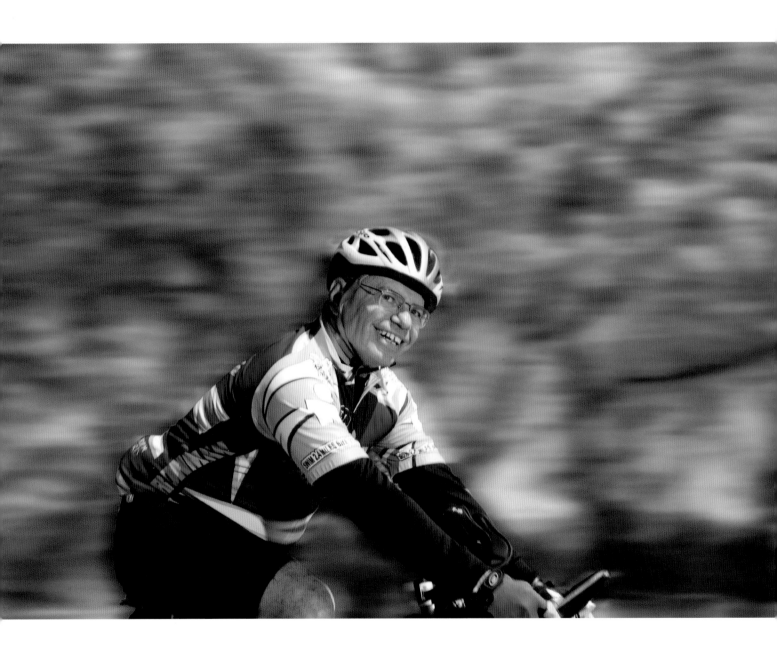

Haim Geffen

Retired Transportation Planner
Age at diagnosis, 53
Colorectal cancer, 2000
Open heart surgery, 2010

Thirty-five years ago, I became a triathlete and a marathon runner. Twenty-five years ago I became a vegetarian, eating mostly fruits and vegetables. And then in 2000, I got cancer. I was shocked because I thought I had been protecting myself. It made me realize that no one is immune. I decided to take it one day at a time.

After I got over the initial shock, I went through a long process of information gathering and learning. There are a lot of decisions to make and no frame of reference when you start. I mostly needed someone to tell me what it's like to go through this. I felt like I was in a vacuum. My doctor told me that I had five options for treatment. I had no idea what to choose. I did not understand why I was the one who had to choose.

I'm now busier than I ever was when I was working. Cancer became a stimulus for me to start thinking about my retirement, doing things I like to do, and helping other people. I now visit nursing homes and I'm an advocate for the aging. I am also leading a support group for newly diagnosed cancer patients. Sharing both my cancer experience and my ability to continue my previous lifestyle is rewarding because I can see how it gives newly diagnosed patients hope.

A few years after my diagnosis, I had to have angioplasty and a shunt put in my heart. Two months after that, I did a 100-mile bike ride. I continued to train by riding and running on my own. Around this time, I did a bike race with a six-mile run afterward. Because I had fairly bad fatigue as a side effect from one of my medications, I barely finished and came in last. But I won first place because I was the only person in my age group. That race is just like having cancer. All you have to do is finish the race to be a winner.

In 2010 I had a new challenge. Due to the progression of my heart disease, I went through a double bypass, open-heart surgery. Again, I had to start rebuilding my body and mind from a low point and rekindle my passion, the triathlon. A year later, at the age of sixty-five, I participated in another Ironman distance triathlon. This time I saw myself as a winner just to make it to the starting line.

I have lists of things I want to do that I have never done. We all have a limited time on earth, so we should make it the most meaningful and enjoy it.

We all have a limited time on earth, so we should make it the most meaningful and enjoy it.

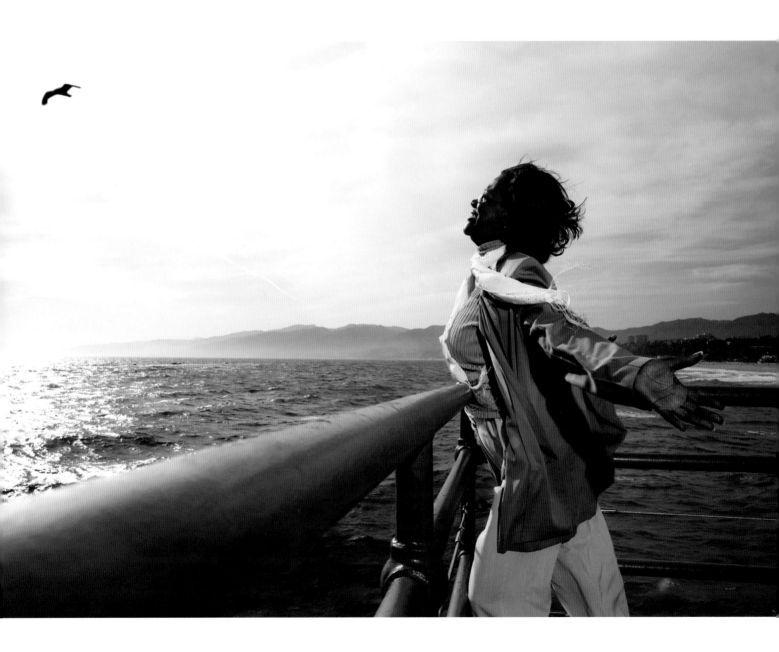

Hazel Madison

Age at first diagnosis, 48
Hodgkin's lymphoma,
Metastasized to brain and spine, 1994

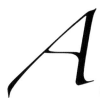 fter I was diagnosed, I had just about come to the conclusion that life was not worth living any longer. I was not even sure if I wanted the brain surgery that my doctor was so adamantly insisting on. And then I met a seventy-two-year-old man who took care of me. He was a former addiction counselor, and he knew what it was like to not want to live. He stayed with me in the beginning, and then we finally "jumped the broom" to make it legal.

Now I am so much smarter. I know how to take care of myself, and I know how to say no.

A lot of people, including my family, used to tell me I was ugly. Then one day a good friend said, "You are not ugly. Stop letting people tell you that." Now I feel good about myself; I feel beautiful. My body is changing for the better, and feelings of intimacy are coming back.

Today I love everything: the trees, the flowers, even people who give me the finger. I have started to think, *Maybe I can help others.*

> *Today I love everything: the trees, the flowers, even people who give me the finger.*

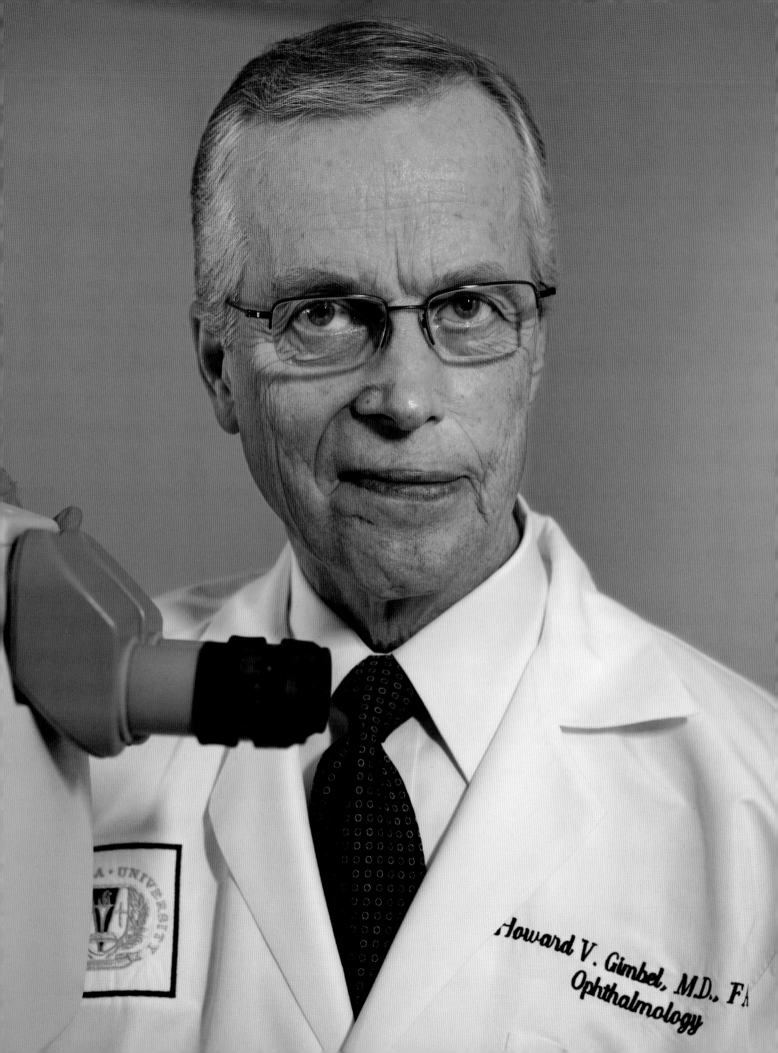

Howard Gimbel, MD

Master of Public Health, Fellow of the
Royal College of Surgeons,
American College of Surgeons
Age at first diagnosis, 66
Prostate cancer, 2000
Sclerosing Basal cell carcinoma, 2000
Perineural Basal cell carcinoma, 2005

*D*uring my first cancer, I kept working all through my treatments. I breezed right through it. I had my treatments at 7:00 a.m. and was at work at 8:00 a.m. I was so pleased with the outcome that it was almost a nonevent for me.

About the same time, I had another diagnosis. A dermatologist found sclerosing basal cell carcinoma on my face. That also was repaired and taken care of, but about five years later, I had numbness and tingling on the side of my nose. No doctor had seen anything like it. Eventually, I found a doctor in Florida who was convinced it was perineural basal cell carcinoma.

So I had to go back to proton treatments once again. By now, I knew the path to the proton accelerator quite well, and went down for another forty treatments. With God's help in letting it heal on its own, I didn't need plastic surgery.

I had been on the board of a university when we were struggling with spending $40 million on unproven proton treatment. Little did I realize that my life would be saved by it, not once, but twice.

All along these diagnoses and treatments, my wife and I didn't get emotional. It was just something that had to be done. My outlook on life helped me take it in stride. If it was going to be fatal, I felt that I'd had a very fulfilling life with no regrets, only thankfulness. It strengthened my faith, and I always had the conviction that nothing is impossible for God. He could cure it, or he might elect that it run its course. I was okay with every option. Now I thank Him that He chose to preserve my life.

> *I value and treasure being healthy and alive. And because I've recovered from two cancers, I feel doubly blessed.*

I also know that our nutrition discipline has enhanced our lifestyle and our health. My wife is so good to me in how she cooks for me for every meal.

I value and treasure being healthy and alive. And because I've recovered from two cancers, I feel doubly blessed.

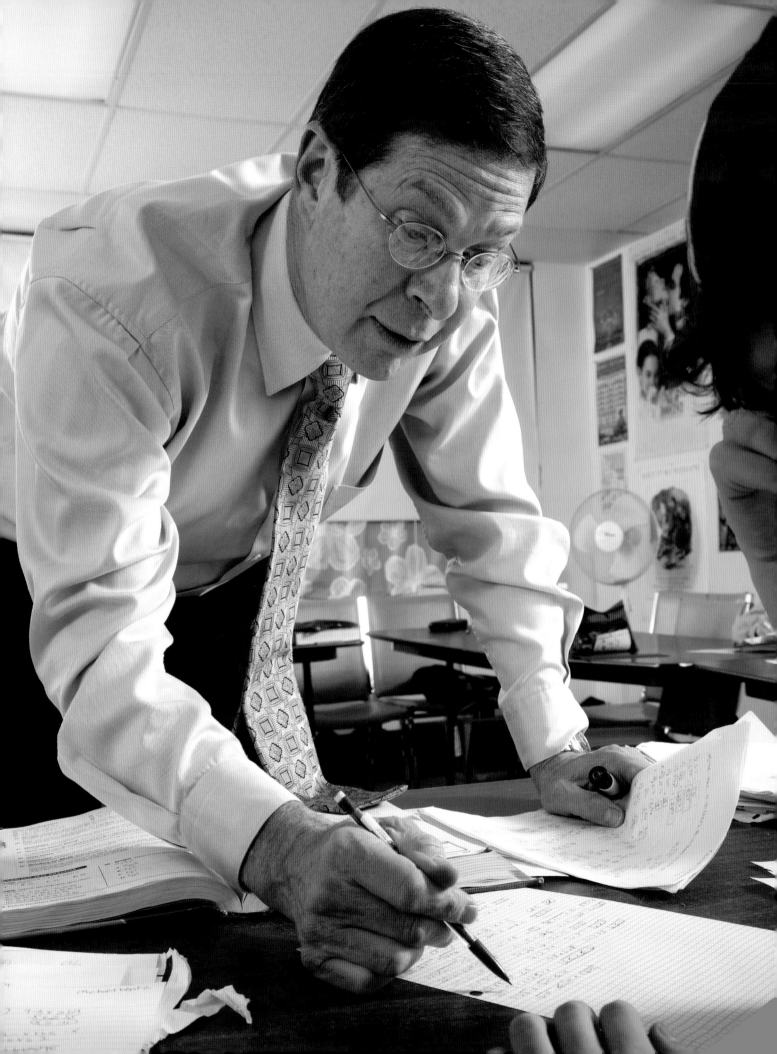

Howard Mendelson, MD

Pediatrician, Math Teacher
Age at first diagnosis, 31
Colon cancer, 1980
Testicular cancer, 1989

*T*he first time around, cancer didn't change my life. My life was good; I just had a little medical setback. It annoyed me because I had things to do with my life. I couldn't be bothered with illness.

Developing a second cancer, one of a different type, less than ten years after the first one affected me more profoundly. I began to question the importance of so many aspects of my life. I became much more selective about what I tolerated. A colleague told me that one day he looked at his career and at his ratio of *"nachis* to *narishkite,"* which means joy to nonsense. That was so profound for me, because after two cancers, I no longer had any tolerance for nonsense.

> *. . . after two cancers, I no longer had any tolerance for nonsense.*

What was important was life and family. I had the chance of having them ripped out from under me twice. I realized the balance was upside down. I was burnt-out professionally and did not want to spend time doing something that no longer gave me joy. I walked away from a very lucrative practice without a plan. Why earn a lot of money and be unhappy? It seemed crazy. And yet, I loved being busy and productive all the time.

During all my years in practice as a pediatrician, I tutored children in math and science. It was very common to have high school or college students come over to my house after dinner so I could help them. Many times, I couldn't wait to finish my clinical practice to get home and tutor for free. I knew there was something wrong with that picture.

I knew I loved tutoring and working with children. I asked a friend about a teaching opportunity for high school math, and shortly thereafter began a second profession. After a few months, I already knew I loved it. To this day, I still do. It is personally very satisfying, and I make incredible bonds with the kids and their parents.

My encounters with cancer have given me the time to reflect on what is really important in my life, make some directional changes in careers, and most important, has helped me to once again find joy in a meaningful profession.

Jackie Martinoski

Sales Manager
Age at diagnosis, 37
Colon cancer, stage 4, 2006
Recurrence, 2008
Treatments continuing through 2013

By the time I was diagnosed, my cancer had metastasized to the liver with numerous lesions. The HMO doctors told me that I had three to six months to live, and I wasn't even a candidate for treatment. Even though I was sick and in great pain, I was constantly on the phone with my insurance company. I begged them to cover my tests and surgery and to please give me a chance.

Because of an amazing support system that kept telling me to do research and get other opinions, I found an oncologist at USC Norris Hospital. He told me that there was hope. I'll never forget when he said to me, "I believe I can cure you." My family still calls him "our angel."

I never felt defeated, but at first, just a little overwhelmed, depressed, and in total shock. Then I put myself into "kick cancer's ass" mode. It picked the wrong person to mess with. Never for a minute did I feel like it would get me. I looked at it as a very big inconvenience. I knew I could help myself, but the hardest part was worrying about my family.

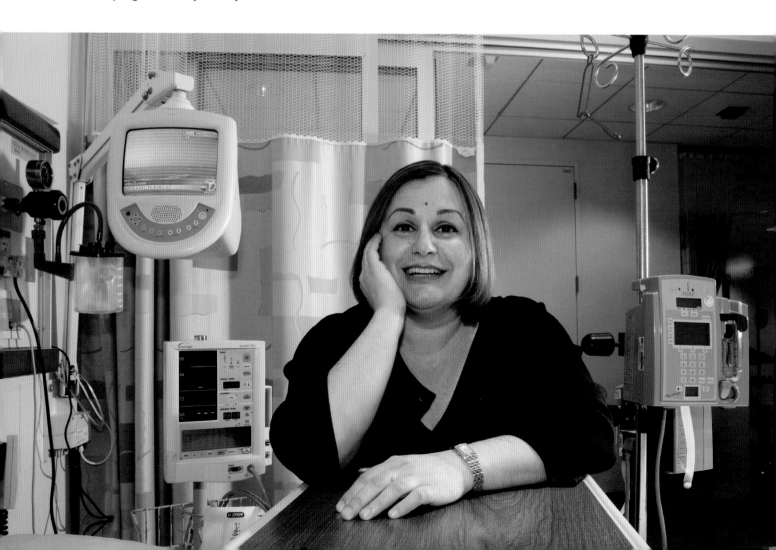

I moved in with my boyfriend in January 2008, and was diagnosed with cancer in March. I told him that I would not be upset if he decided to leave. I would understand. His response was, "You're way too bratty for cancer. Matter of fact, you're such a brat, you can't just get sick; you have to get cancer. Get better and we'll move on."

The hospital called me "the miracle girl." I went into remission for a year and a half, and then I had a recurrence in my liver. I've finished chemo, and more surgeries are planned to remove remaining metastases.

I now know there are a lot of great people out there. I met amazing caretakers and families who were going through difficult challenges. Because I've learned so much, I want to return the same favor. When you get a diagnosis, all you want is a little hope. I can give hope now, and I have to remember to keep giving it to myself. Cancer is by no means a death sentence.

> *I'm going to keep kicking cancer's ass.*

I want to make a difference and eventually become an advocate for people with cancer. I want to speak and motivate and do something positive with my life. Once you get cancer, you will always have a cancer attitude. I want to be like Lance Armstrong, only not famous and not dating Sheryl Crow.

I have a list of so many things I want to do and places I want to see. I'm going to keep kicking cancer's ass.

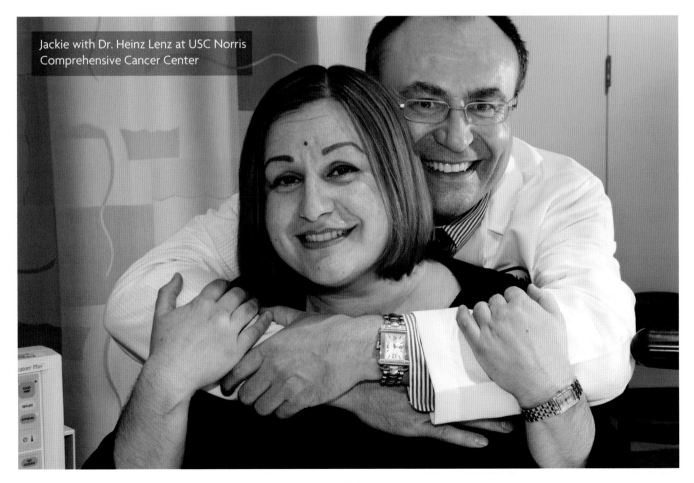

Jackie with Dr. Heinz Lenz at USC Norris Comprehensive Cancer Center

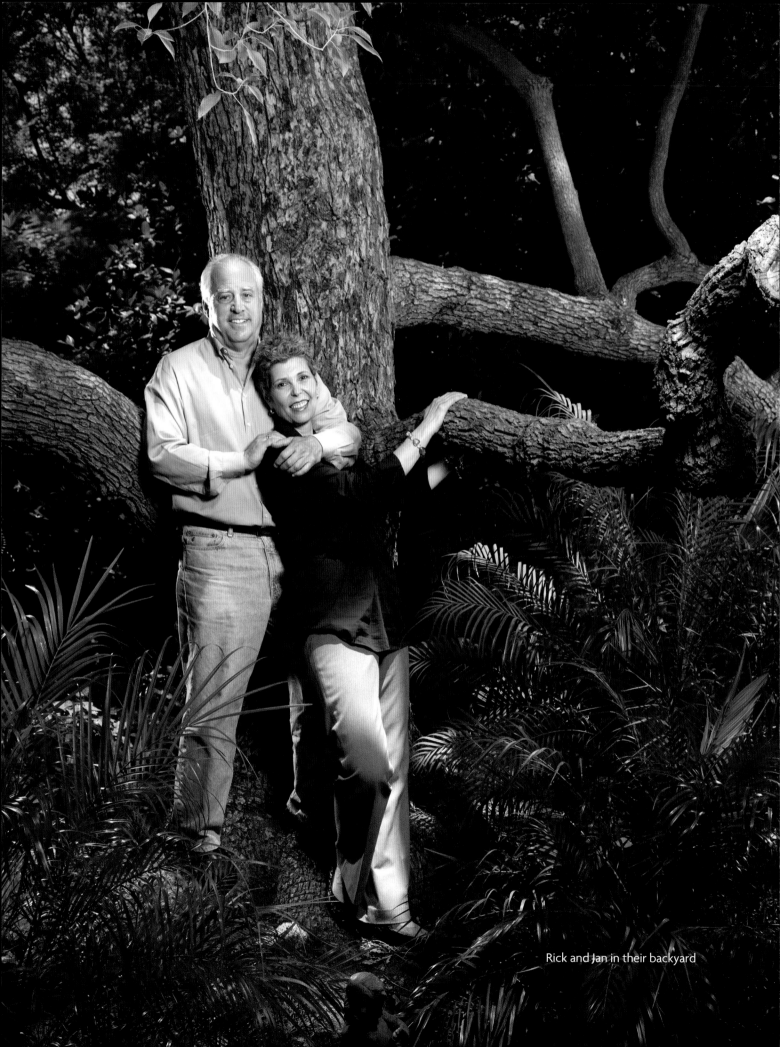

Rick and Jan in their backyard

Jan Platt

Professional Mom and Wife, Event Planner
Breast cancer, 2003
Primary peritoneal and ovarian cancer, 2005
Recurrence, 2007

JAN: I continued to work on my event planning business through the lumpectomy and radiation during my first round of cancer,. The morning after surgery, I was finishing wedding invitations for a nervous bride. That is when my view of life and priorities first began to change.

A year later, I started to notice changes in my body. Things weren't right. When I had a strange reaction at a movie theatre my friend took me directly from the movie to the hospital. After a series of tests, they told me I had too much salt on my popcorn. I continued to get worse, and they eventually discovered I had ovarian cancer. I was numb and paralyzed, but I was way too stubborn to die. My saga began again, but the lessons continued to grow.

The outpouring of help from my family and friends made me realize how much I was loved. The angels in my life couldn't do enough. I learned from them that you don't ask, "What can I do?" You just do something. When I was too sick to take care of my husband and sons, my friends helped do it for me. Because of them, I learned to be a better friend, a better mom, and a better wife.

Humor helps get me through the day. I've only worn a wig eight or ten times. Once was at a wedding, where I didn't want to draw attention to myself. When a woman wanted to know who did my hair, I told her she could easily have the same cut, "Just come in the ladies' room and I'll show you how."

RICK, JAN'S HUSBAND: And she's the prettiest bald woman you've ever seen.

JAN: I don't like how cancer has defined me. Most people still want to whisper the word. They don't know how to approach me. The best way is to simply say, "I know this is a tough time for you. I'm here to listen and help."

The hospital staff has been amazing. You can't put a value on the doctor who holds your hand. And they can't believe how dedicated my husband has been. He is a very sensitive, sweet soul, and he is there for me through everything.

RICK: I have been quickly humbled. I often feel powerless. I've gone from "There's nothing I can't do" to "There's nothing I can do."

JAN: This has made our family closer in so many ways. I always knew they loved me, but I never knew love could be this unconditional. My sons used to keep emotions inside, but not now. I still have a text message my son sent after my third diagnosis: "Mom, you are loved. We'll beat this." I'll never give that phone away.

I have learned to change my priorities and set up boundaries. I am trying to teach myself when to say "no" and when to say "I love you." I used to keep too much inside. Now I let it out. I cry unconditional tears of joy.

Some days I'm not sure I can make it, or if I want to. Then the emotional side of my brain takes over when I look at my husband and children. I have been on six different protocols of chemo spanning six to eight months each. My life has been on constant chemo. I've lost my hair four times. I never thought I would walk down the path of cancer, but I have, and I'm a better, stronger person because of it. I sign all of my letters "I am woman. Hear me roar."

I sign all of my letters "I am woman. Hear me roar."

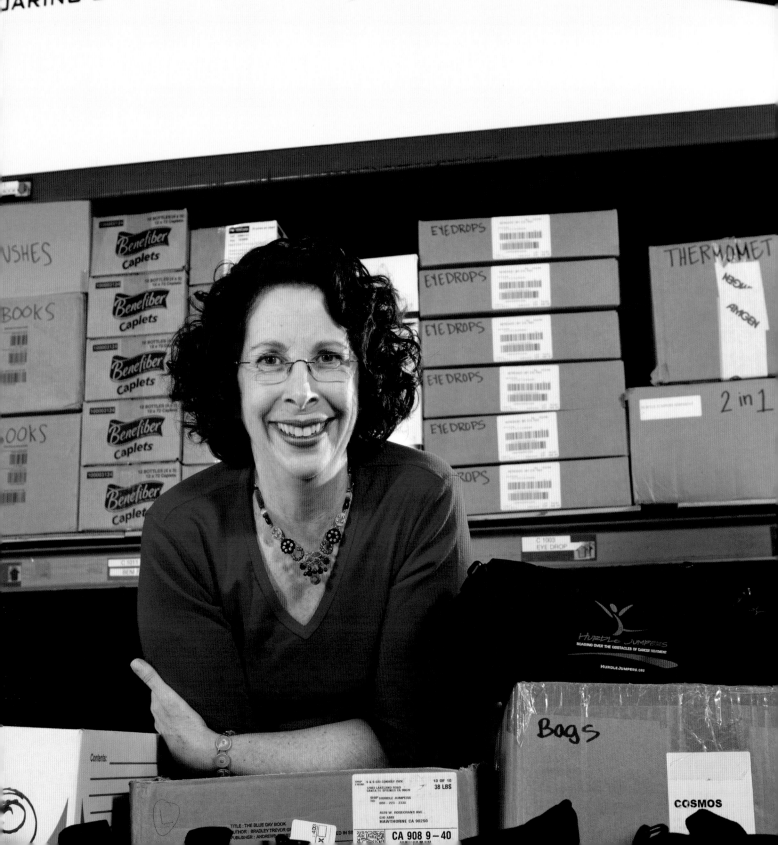

Janet R. Halbert

Business Management Consultant, CPA,
Founder of "Hurdle Jumpers®"
Age at diagnosis, 49
Breast cancer, 2004

I was well aware of the importance of a breast self-exam, so when I felt a lump, I was terrified. A biopsy confirmed it, and I heard those three dreaded words: "You have cancer."

I was only eleven years old when my mother died of breast cancer. When I got my diagnosis thirty-eight years later, I was living my worst nightmare, but I knew it wasn't a death sentence. As it turns out, I didn't have the breast cancer gene, just bad luck. So I embarked on a year of surgery, chemotherapy, and radiation treatments.

Although they try, health-care professionals cannot completely prepare a patient for all the possible side effects of treatment. It was exhausting spending my dwindling energy tracking down products to alleviate symptoms and annoying side effects like dry eyes, dry mouth, skin infection, or stomach distress. As a business consultant, I'm a professional problem solver, and I knew I wanted to solve this problem after I recovered.

> *I'm a professional problem solver, and I knew I wanted to solve this problem after I recovered.*

I often thought about how new mothers leave the hospital with a care kit and wondered why there was no kit for patients with cancer. I wanted to make sure patients, ready to embark on their own journey to wellness, could avoid the frustration and challenges I experienced. I saw an unmet need and created a solution, Hurdle Jumpers' Chemo and Radiation Kits. I named the nonprofit charity Hurdle Jumpers because we help patients with cancer soar over the obstacles of treatment.

Each patient care kit is filled with informative tips; donated consumer health products; practical tools, such as a gentle toothbrush, jar opener, and thermometer; a relaxation CD; and a humor book. The messages of hope and inspiration and a reminder that most side effects are temporary fill the recipient with confidence and powerful knowledge.

It's hard to believe, but a cancer diagnosis gave me a big dose of gratitude. And at Hurdle Jumpers we are so grateful to companies who donate their products, our hundreds of volunteers, and for generous support from the community. We celebrate our success in distributing over four thousand kits in six years, but recently reduced our activities due to financial constraints.

No one is ever the same after any cancer diagnosis. In creating a charity to assist others, it helped me heal from my own emotional roller-coaster ride. I took the lemons of a cancer diagnosis and made lemon meringue pie.

A purposeful life for me is knowing that I've made someone else's life better. I can never go back to the time before my diagnosis, so I have adjusted to a new normal.

I dedicated this charity work to my parents. My mom was diagnosed when cancer was a whispered word, and my dad was her caregiver. At a young age, they taught me an important life skill of giving back. They were truly the first hurdle jumpers in my life.

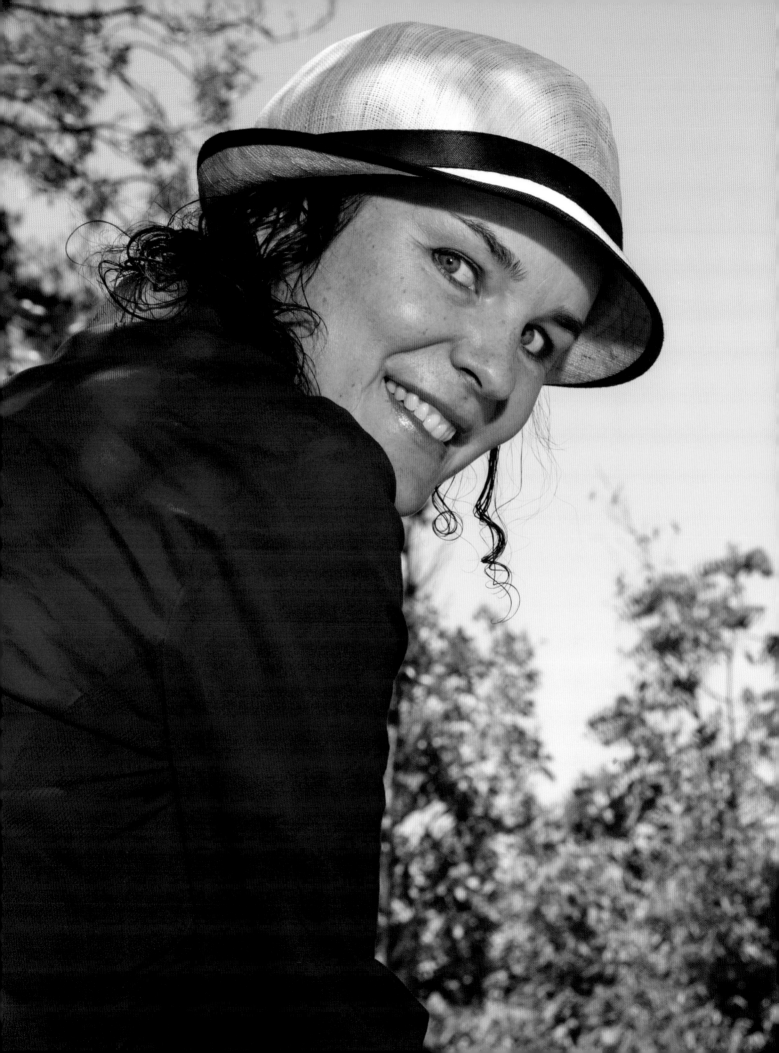

Jeannine Walston

Cancer Coach, Writer, Consultant, Speaker
Age at diagnosis, 24
Oligodendroglioma (Oligo Astrocytoma), 1998
Recurrence, 2000

One day in 1998, while I was working for the US Congress, I felt dizzy. A general practitioner sent me to an ear doctor who ordered an MRI, which revealed a brain tumor. I was twenty-four years old; my world suddenly collapsed into an existence of fear and uncertainty.

I researched options and chose the National Institutes of Health to perform awake brain surgery. One month later after returning to work, parts of me felt extremely different. In a world turned upside down, I began to learn some strategies for my optimal wellness. I used complementary treatments, alternative therapies, and self-care for body, mind, and spirit. I put aside my plans for law school and in 2000 began working for cancer nonprofits and as a consultant to the National Cancer Institute and Food and Drug Administration.

Ultimately I realized the importance of not only focusing on the disease but also of addressing the whole person, both personally and professionally. In order to heal, I wanted to find answers as I struggled to transform myself. The National Center for Complementary and Alternative Medicine hired me but, once again, I became sick in the summer of 2003—this time with Epstein-Barr virus and chronic fatigue syndrome—and had to leave my job.

In early 2004, I learned I had another recurrence. As it turns out, the MRI scans revealed that the tumors had actually returned in 2000. By 2011, I needed to undergo a second awake brain surgery at UCSF, and a third one at UCLA in 2013. Since then, I have had radiation plus oral chemotherapy and a clinical trial of dendritic cell vaccines with immunotherapy.

> *I encourage the spirit of self-awareness, which, as I discovered, can lead to true happiness.*

Cancer presents many challenges: physically, emotionally, and often financially. During my own stages of intense chaos and confusion, I experienced major improvements from mind-body wellness strategies, self-awareness, love and support, and my soul's spiritual evolution.

I am now a "Cancer Coach," helping cancer patients and their caregivers with integrative treatments that address the mind, body, and soul. My hope is that the inspiration and information I provide will help those affected by cancer to evolve, transform, and heal. I encourage the spirit of self-awareness, which, as I discovered, can lead to true happiness.

Jenee Areeckal

Social Worker
Age at first diagnosis, 15
Osteogenic sarcoma, January 1985
Recurrence in the lungs, May 1985
Recurrence in the heart, 1988
Ovarian cancer, 2008

I was fifteen years old and living in Spain with my family when I discovered a bump on my knee. That bump turned out to be bone cancer. I had two options: fusing my knee or amputating my leg. Thanks to my orthopedic surgeon, I was able to meet an amputee mentor, who used a prosthesis. It became clear to me that amputation was the better option. Fusing my knee would prohibit me from playing sports and would make it difficult to travel. Amputation also seemed to be a good way of getting rid of the cancer in hopes that it would never return.

Four months after amputation, my worst nightmare occurred; the cancer had metastasized in my lungs. The doctors informed my parents that I had three months to live. But after one and a half years of chemotherapy, radiation seeds placed in my lungs, and two lung surgeries, I went into remission. Life was back to normal. I went back to school, finished my senior year, graduated, and began college.

Life was good for another year and a half. Then, once again, life threw me another curve ball. I relapsed for the second time, this time in my heart. I was eighteen years old and already I had experienced cancer twice. I had a

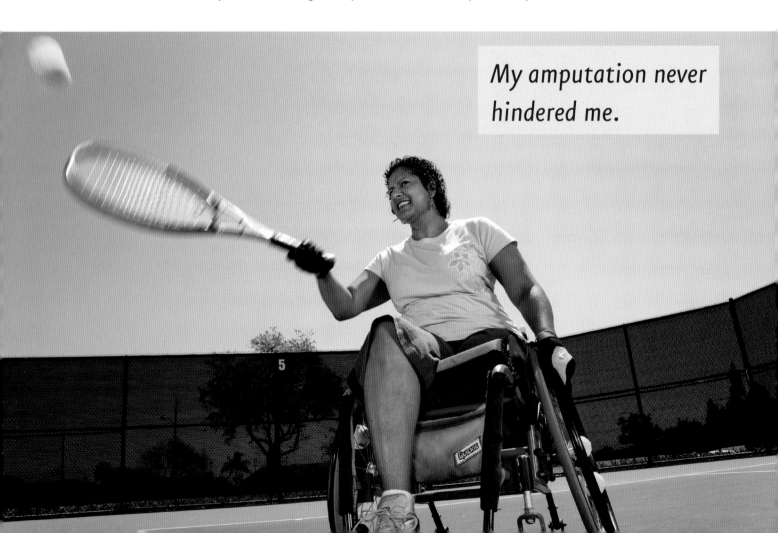

My amputation never hindered me.

5

hard time adjusting back into the role of an active cancer patient; doctors planned an open heart surgery and another year of chemotherapy. I was very angry with God.

I finished my bachelor's degree in sociology, and then years later a master's in social work. I got my dream job in pediatric oncology, where I help children, teens, and their families with that initial diagnosis of cancer. I provide that positive energy of never giving up, which helps lower their anxiety. In the Indian culture, it is difficult to talk about emotions and disabilities, so I understand how hard the fight can be with some families.

I still ski and swim, and I recently started playing tennis again in a wheelchair.

In 2008 I was diagnosed with ovarian cancer. Once again I had to put all my emotions on hold and fight. This battle was truly the hardest for me because it came with a loss of the ability to have children. I had a girlfriend who died, but she taught me to live in the moment, because that moment will never come again. You never know what will happen tomorrow. This is what I pass on to my patients and their families.

Cancer survivors either break or develop a very thick skin. I know that my strength and my humor pulled me through every time. People, particularly men, are often intimidated by me. They have to accept my prosthetic leg along with me. Humor has always helped in getting others more relaxed with my leg. I tell people there are no stupid questions.

My ultimate goal is to have a camp for amputee children that would include sports, meditation, self-reflection, and self-esteem. It is important to help them be strong, to show them how to deal with all that they have lost, and to let them know that they can lead a normal life. My amputation never hindered me. I did all the things a normal teenage girl would do. I still ski and swim, and I recently started playing tennis again in a wheelchair.

My hope is that I have become an example so that everyone becomes comfortable with amputees and the disabled. I know I have one leg up on everyone else.

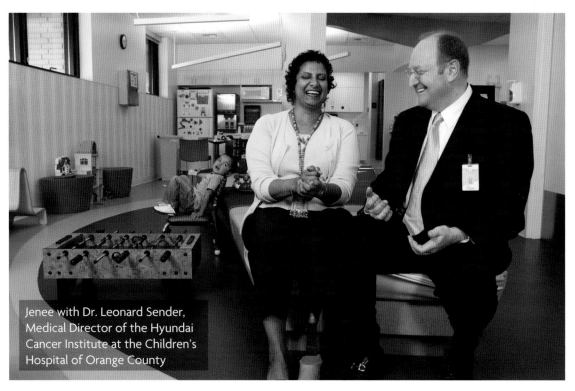

Jenee with Dr. Leonard Sender, Medical Director of the Hyundai Cancer Institute at the Children's Hospital of Orange County

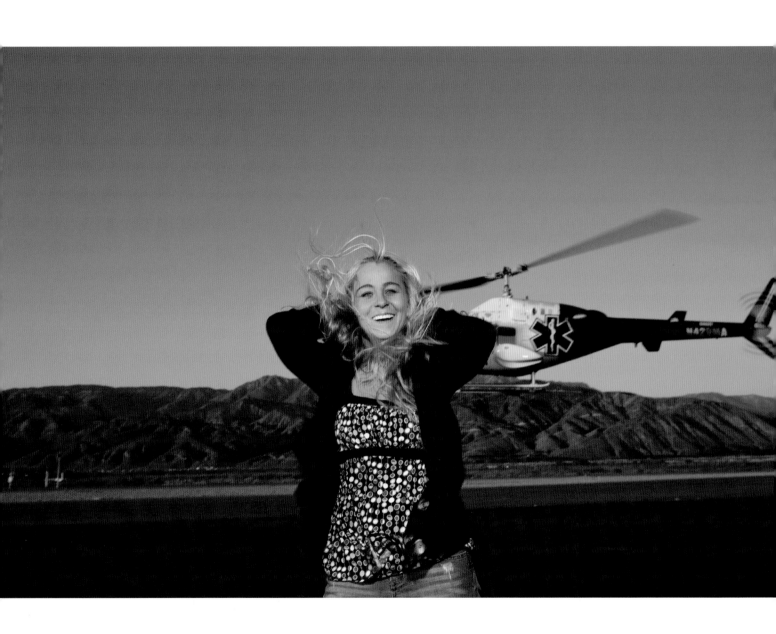

Jennifer Gardner

Paramedic, Life Flight Student
Age at diagnosis, 16
Astrocytoma brain tumor, 1997

I was a sixteen-year-old cross-country runner and hurdler, and my only worry was what date I was going to take to the prom. Then the doctors discovered a tumor behind my eyes. I made my brother promise me that he would tell me right away after the surgery if it was cancer. He told me that if I had to fight cancer, he would buy me a truck. As I woke up from the surgery, my whole family was there. My brother said, "It's cancer," and the very first thing I said was, "Four by four?"

But it was bad. The doctors found out the cancer had spread all through my brain and that there was nothing they could do. I had about four months to live.

I refused to listen to them. There was no way I was going to let cancer beat me. I think there are two kinds of people: those who give up and those who don't. I've seen both sides, and I can only think about being on one side. That said, if it weren't for my family kicking my butt, I wouldn't have made it. I have five brothers and sisters, and we became a very close family because of this. I was so scared, and yet the experience was awesome because of them and my new family of doctors and nurses.

> *There was no way I was going to let cancer beat me.*

I went through nine surgeries and proton radiation. I didn't pray to live and I didn't pray to die. I just prayed for God to show me His will. I vowed to share his testimony. Now He has proven to me that His will is better than anything I could have planned. It sounds weird, but I am thankful for my cancer; I feel like I lucked out getting it.

Because I conquered cancer, I proved to myself that if I want something, no matter what, I can get it. I would never have the passion that I have today without first having had that experience. Now it seems normal to go after anything I want. God gave me cancer, and cancer gave me opportunity.

I would never have even thought about going into the medical field. Now my biggest joy in life is helping other people. I would not have said that before cancer. I was shallow and snotty.

I love working in flight operations. I also take Homeland Security classes, because I was so inspired after 9/11. And I'm a surfer, an adrenaline junkie. I love staying busy. As strange as it sounds, I get an adrenaline rush when helping people, and that's what saves their lives.

I love life. That is one thing that I know for certain.

> *I love life. That is one thing that I know for certain.*

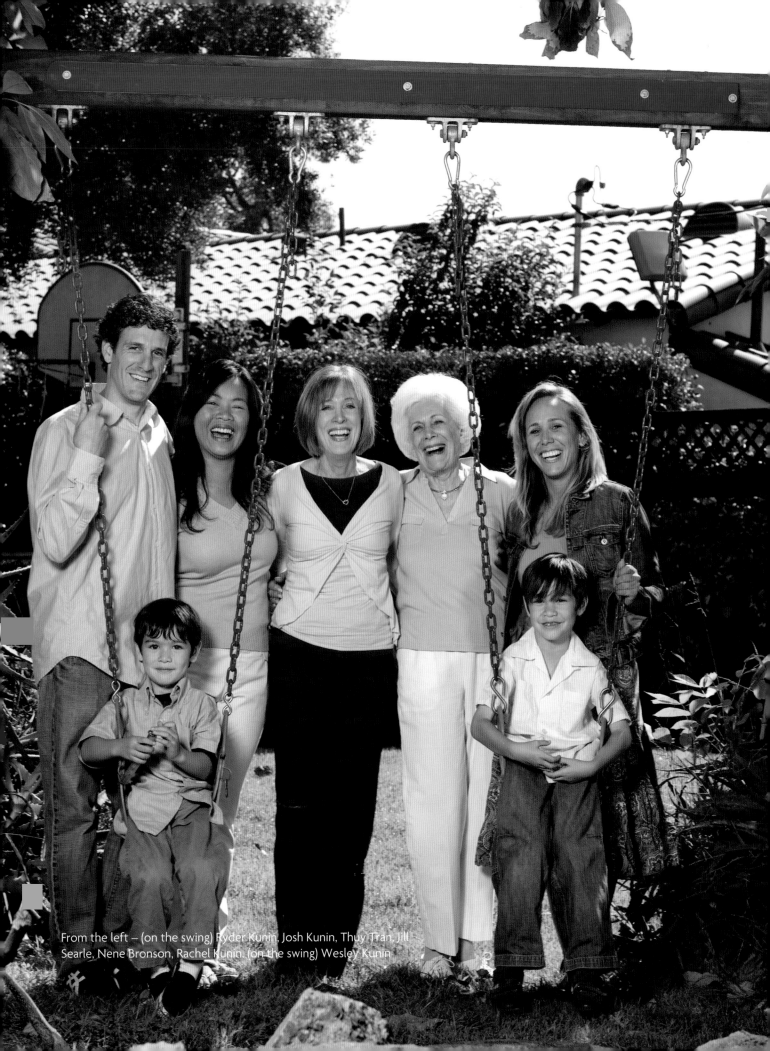

From the left – (on the swing) Ryder Kunin, Josh Kunin, Thuy Tran, Jill Searle, Nene Bronson, Rachel Kunin, (on the swing) Wesley Kunin

Jill Searle

Psychotherapist, Clinical Program Director, Cancer Support Community—Pasadena
Age at diagnosis, 41
Breast cancer, 1987

*I*n 1987 when I was diagnosed with breast cancer, I was relatively young. My children were teenagers at the time, and I wondered throughout my treatment whether I would be there to celebrate the milestones of their lives—graduations, career decisions, weddings, the birth of their children. I recognize that I have been fortunate beyond measure to have both survived and thrived.

After my experience with cancer, I knew that I wanted to do something with my life wherein I could use my intelligence and my experience for a greater good. I didn't know what that would look like until years later when I decided to go back to school to pursue a master's degree in psychology and a license in marriage and family therapy. As part of my training, I became an intern at what is now the Cancer Support Community. I found that working with people affected by cancer has given meaning to my own experience.

> *After my experience with cancer, I knew that I wanted to do something with my life . . .*

Being a program director and group facilitator has been a way for me to bring it full circle—to pay it forward, if you will. I am immensely gratified that I can be there for someone newly diagnosed and likely quite scared, and that I can bring with me a story of survival and hope.

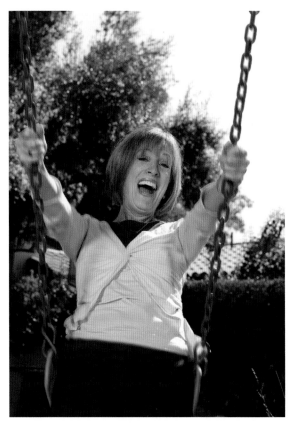

115

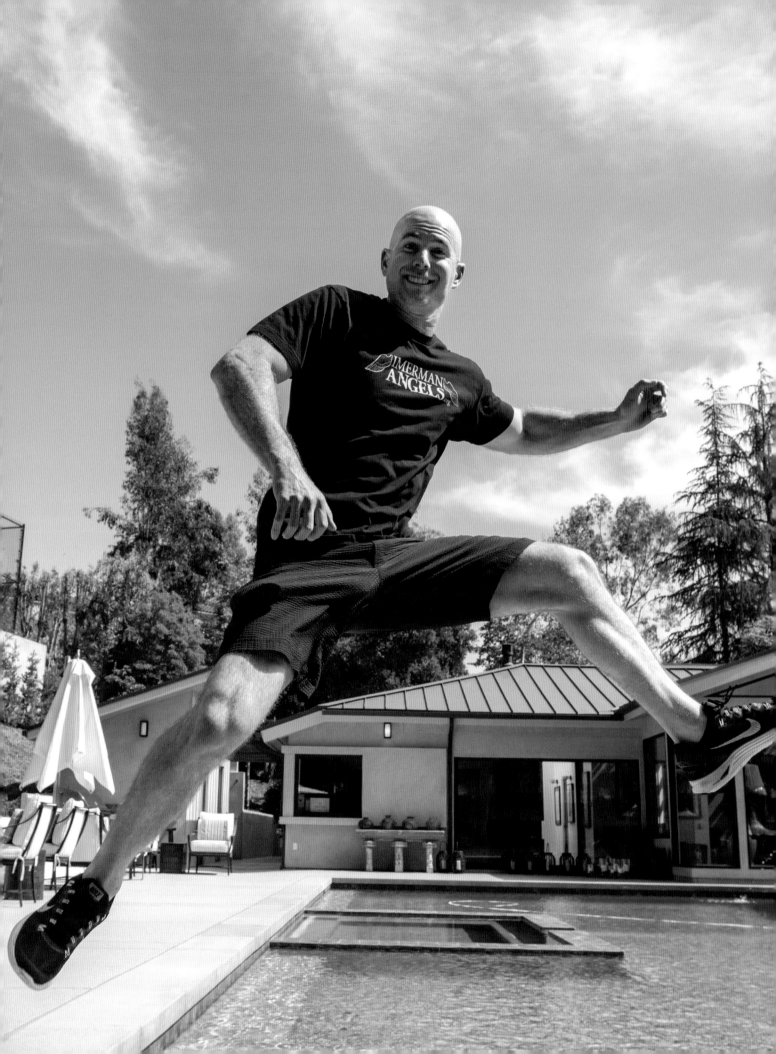

Jonny Imerman

Chief Mission Officer, Imerman Angels
Age at diagnosis, 26
Testicular cancer, 2002

I was diagnosed with testicular cancer in 2002 when I was twenty-six years old. At that age, you aren't thinking about health challenges; you're thinking about the gym, building a career, and feeling healthy. I was having fun in a bar one night with friends when I had the worst possible pain. I dropped the pool stick and doubled over. I pretended I was fine, waddled to my car, drove myself to the hospital, and found out the news that would change my life forever.

I was tired and nauseous most of the time for nearly six months when I went through surgery and chemo. Every time I looked in the mirror, I cried. My confidence was zero point zero. Slowly, I began to heal and feel better, and then, a year later, they found four tumors behind my kidneys along my spine. They removed my organs, took out the tumors, and then put all my organs back in my body with more than sixty staples. I prayed to God that, if I lived, I would give back to the world for my life.

More important than any personal story, I believe, is the challenge to think about what we can do to help other people. How do we allow this experience to inspire us? I knew that there had to be many people still on the other side who needed my friendship. Two weeks after my last chemo, before the recurrence, I told my doctors that I wanted to help motivate young, newly diagnosed cancer patients. I started going room-to-room, door-to-door, introducing myself. Cancer is an emotional time when the world stops, and all you think about is getting your life back. People want to talk, particularly young people to young people.

> *More important than any personal story, I believe, is the challenge to think about what we can do to help other people.*

I did that on nights and weekends for years, never believing it would eventually become a career. I quit my job in real estate when I was twenty-nine. People started donating time and money, and that's when I realized it was something that the world needed. I began building a database of survivors and connecting them with patients one-on-one. I soon started getting stories from all over the country. Today Imerman Angels has 6,000 survivors and caregivers worldwide in more than sixty countries and a staff of ten full-time people. The snowball found its own path.

There are many cancer patients fighting their disease on one side of the river and millions of happy survivors on the other side. I like to think that we are building a bridge to connect them.

I've been good now for more than ten years. I never dreamed that I would be running an organization of this kind, the largest in the world. When you're diagnosed and going through treatment, you're never thinking two steps ahead. You're thinking one inch in front of you. We hope to make the path brighter, clearer, easier and faster. We want to change lives.

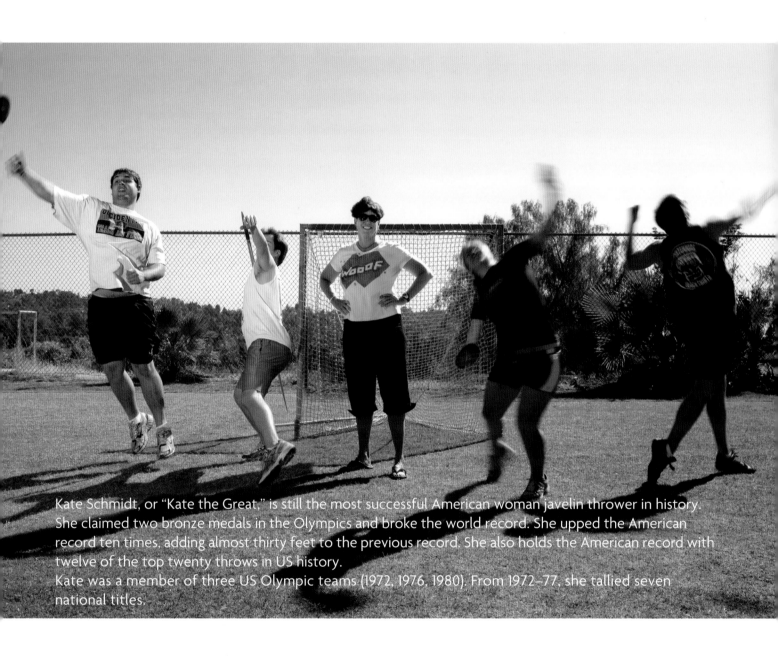

Kate Schmidt, or "Kate the Great," is still the most successful American woman javelin thrower in history. She claimed two bronze medals in the Olympics and broke the world record. She upped the American record ten times, adding almost thirty feet to the previous record. She also holds the American record with twelve of the top twenty throws in US history.

Kate was a member of three US Olympic teams (1972, 1976, 1980). From 1972–77, she tallied seven national titles.

Kate Schmidt

Olympian, Track and Field Coach
Age at diagnosis, 39
Ovarian cancer, 1993

*I*n August of 1993, I went on a camping trip with a good friend and my dog, Bubba. While sitting around the campfire, Bubba jumped in my lap and began pawing at my stomach. I had been in pain, and so that intrigued me. The next day I went to the hospital and found out that I had a burst tumor right where Bubba sensed it. I was diagnosed with stage 1C aggressive ovarian cancer.

A week later, a woman told me, "You know everyone is terminal." Surprisingly, those words made me feel some relief. It sort of uncorked me to realize that we cannot choose the manner or the time of our deaths. I now have less fear of death because I had the opportunity to face it. Through that period, I never thought I would die. In fact, I was less afraid of dying than I was of the morphine drip. I was six years sober at the time, and I wanted to stay that way. I'm still sober now, for more than twenty-five years.

Now I just take whatever comes. It will be what it is, and that's good. I pray to keep my heart open to whatever is next, because I don't want to miss anything that is placed in front of me.

I don't want to miss anything that is placed in front of me.

I was with a private-training client one day at a local high school, and the track coach told me about an opening for another coaching position, something I never thought I would do. I grabbed it. I thought I better start sharing my knowledge. I taught there for about seventeen years, and then stopped to spend more time enjoying life and being with friends.

As much as possible, I spend time with those I love, and I don't hang around people I don't like. My therapist tells me I'm really good with the big stuff. It's the daily living stuff that I have trouble with.

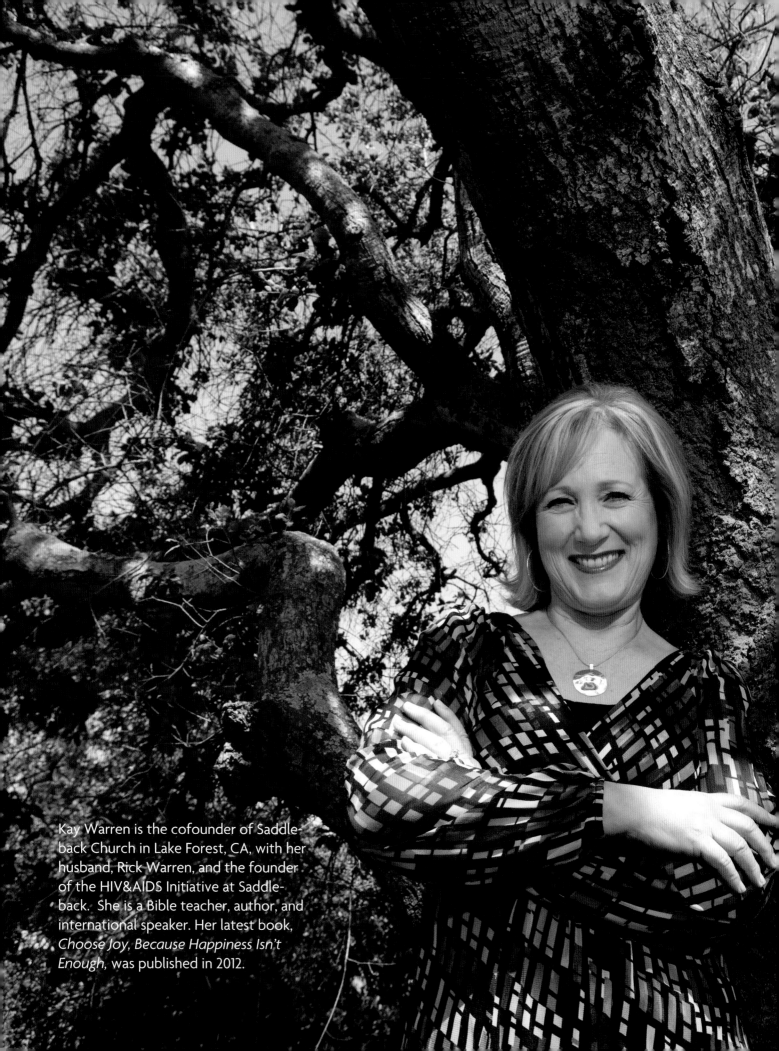

Kay Warren is the cofounder of Saddle-
back Church in Lake Forest, CA, with her
husband, Rick Warren, and the founder
of the HIV&AIDS Initiative at Saddle-
back. She is a Bible teacher, author, and
international speaker. Her latest book,
*Choose Joy, Because Happiness Isn't
Enough,* was published in 2012.

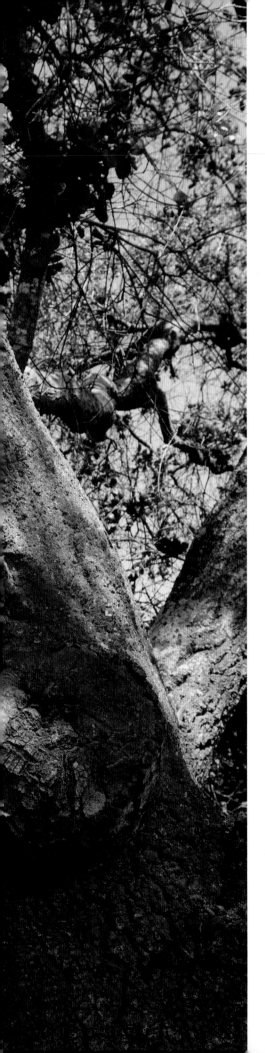

Kay Warren

Age at diagnosis, 49
Breast cancer, 2003
Melanoma, 2005

Cancer shattered my illusion that I have a long life ahead of me. I may. I may not. I can't control how long I live, but I can control *how* I live. One of my mottoes has become "control the controllable and leave the uncontrollable to God." I don't get to determine the number of my days, but I can determine the quality of the days given to me.

The most powerful thing you can do for a person is to simply be with them. Sometimes we just need an arm around our shoulders. For me, it came down to the people in my life who let me question. Nobody rejected me for my thoughts. They stayed with me and represented God to me. I was confused and I didn't understand. It was as if I was pounding on God's chest and asking, "Why are you doing this to me?" I couldn't drive Him away from me. I couldn't make Him let go. Finally I stopped pounding and leaned on Him and cried.

I can't control how long I live, but I can control how I live.

I never got to the place where I didn't think God was real or my faith was shattered. He was real, but I didn't understand His ways or His thought process. Doubt. That was my crisis.

Not only did cancer teach me about suffering on a personal level, it also taught me about the blessings hidden in the suffering. I became aware of how fragile life is, how brief and how holy it is. Knowing life's fragility causes me to be more intentional, more passionate, more convinced of the sweetness of this moment, and more certain than ever before that I am here for a reason. I don't want to waste a second of the time I have been given.

Having cancer a second time just reinforced my determination to live my life very intentionally with no wasted moments. It was another clarion call to fulfill God's purposes with the time I am given. I am determined to live my life, without looking over my shoulder to see if cancer is catching up with me. I want to live for what matters.

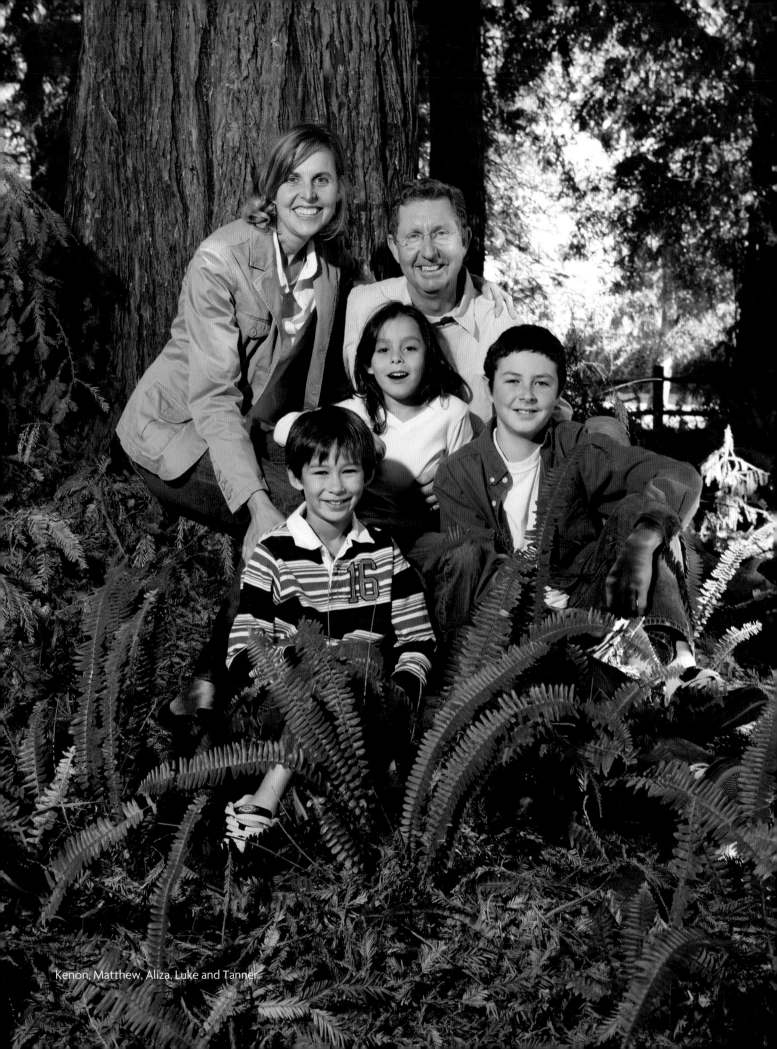

Kenon, Matthew, Aliza, Luke and Tanner

Kenon Neal

Director of Foundation Relations for Westmont College
Age at first diagnosis, 21
Hodgkin's lymphoma, 1987
Recurrence, 1989
Myelodysplasia and bone marrow transplant, 1992
Breast cancer, 2006
Esophageal cancer, 2012
Recurrence (esophageal cancer), 2013
Metastasis in liver and stomach, 2014

KENON: It was just before my senior year in college when I found a lump on my neck. My mom is a laboratory scientist who studies cancer, so she sent me to a hematologist. The doctor immediately knew it was Hodgkin's. In those days, they did surgery and radiation. I sailed through that and even went back to college in the fall.

A year and a half later, I found out it was recurring, so I had an intense new protocol. They were trying to keep me alive, but my body was having trouble keeping up with it. I had to switch treatments.

My husband-to-be stuck with me through everything. When he proposed to me, I was completely bald. He had a great sense of humor and kept me laughing. My doctor gave me three weeks off chemo for a wedding and honeymoon. I put on a wig, tucked my chemo catheter under my wedding dress, and we were off to the church.

MATTHEW, KENON'S HUSBAND: You have to roll with the punches and realize that you don't always get what you want. The idea of leaving a relationship because there was a trial was not part of my worldview. There are never any guarantees. Nothing in me ever said, "Go find something else." There would be no guarantees with that either. I'm just not wired to say that I'll tackle some challenges but not others.

KENON: I was fine for about a year, but my blood counts kept getting worse. I eventually needed a bone marrow transplant in 1993. After that, I had a couple of life-threatening infections, but I slowly built myself back up.

I am thankful for all the opportunities God is giving me to extend life. And for joyful living in the days I am given.

We so badly wanted a family, but because of my past treatments, I was infertile. So we started the adoption process. Each one of my three children has been such a huge blessing in our lives. My oldest son, Tanner, is Hispanic, Russian, and Native American. Luke is half Filipino and half Caucasian, and Aliza is half Native American, half Caucasian. We have a family that is even better than we ever dreamed.

I was in remission for thirteen years and then was diagnosed with breast cancer. This time, with a husband and three children, I was bringing more people with me on the journey. But I knew God would be present.

I was diagnosed last fall with esophageal cancer (due to past radiation) with metastasis to the liver. I went through more chemo and targeted radiation. I am now living scan to scan and God is giving our family strength. It is not an easy road, but we are feeling God's presence as we work through it.

I have always tried to use my experience to encourage others who are going through cancer. They might see it as an ending, but for me it has always been a starting place, a jumping-off place. It enhances my appreciation for everything I do. For most people, having a family is normal; for us, it is extraordinary.

I will always remember the time when my three-year-old daughter was in Bible class learning about people who were bold and courageous. She came running home and said, "Today we learned all about people just like you, people who are bald and courageous."

During my latest round of tests, as the nurse was reading my history, she said, "You are brave." "Well," I replied, "I will be here exactly the number of days that God has planned, not one more or less. That encourages me." I believe in the power of prayer. I know God gives us the strength to walk the journey He carves out before us. I am thankful for all the opportunities God is giving me to extend life. And for joyful living in the days I am given.

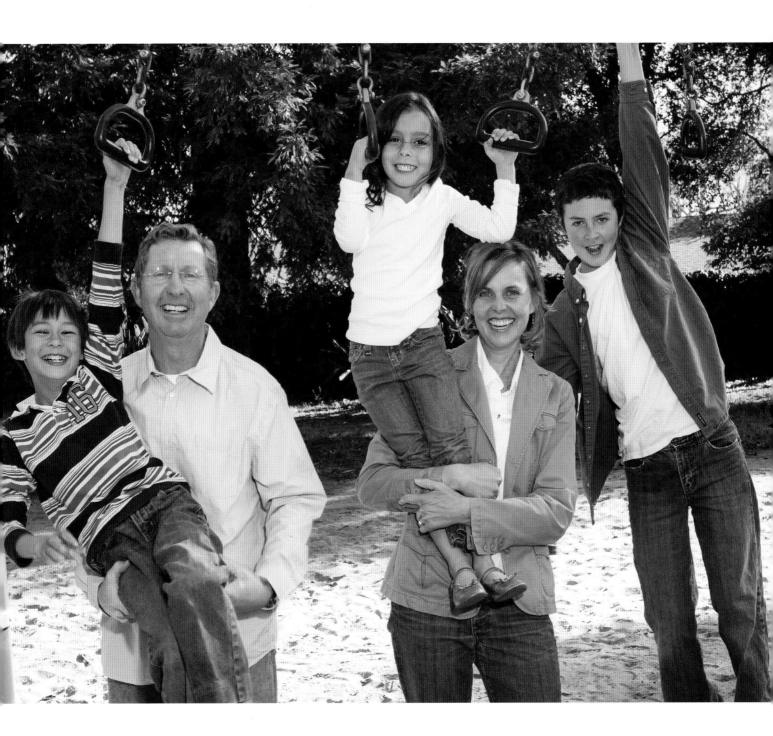

Kevin Carlberg

Musician
Age at diagnosis, 26
Glioblastoma multiforme, grade 4, 2003

A *Rolling Stone* magazine competition had just voted our group the best college band in America, and we were touring in Colorado. During that time, I started having terrible headaches. Then, all of a sudden, doctors told me I had a brain tumor the size of a fist and needed surgery.

I was scared out of my mind, no pun intended. I never thought I would die, but I was worried that I would wake up and not know my fiancée.

We kept our wedding date for two months later, but we downsized it and made it much more intimate. My wife is amazing; she is my rock. I never would have been able to do any of this without her; and because of her, I kept fighting. My daughter, Lyric, is now three years old. Every night the three of us read from a little prayer book, and then she said a prayer for "Daddy's head."

I have a lot more things to do here. I ran the LA Marathon to raise money for the UCLA neurosurgery department. I recently was accepted by an organization called "Love Hope Strength" to do a concert on top of Mount Kilimanjaro. I'm training for the climb now.

My wife reminds me that life is just like training for a marathon. One mile at a time, every day. We make it work, and we can only hope that we inspire others. I have a special T-shirt that I wear when I visit hospitals. It says, "Don't Worry. Be Happy." I want to show patients that there is always hope.

No one is going to tell me when my time is up. I have found out that I am about six times past the length of time they expected me to live, so I've already proven statistics wrong.

> No one is going to tell me when my time is up.

After my surgery, they were shining a bright light into my eyes to wake me up. That light is so symbolic because my life changed right then. I would never say to anyone, "Go get brain surgery; it'll change your life," but it has given me a whole new appreciation. I don't take even the little things for granted, and every morning I say, "Thank you. I'm here again."

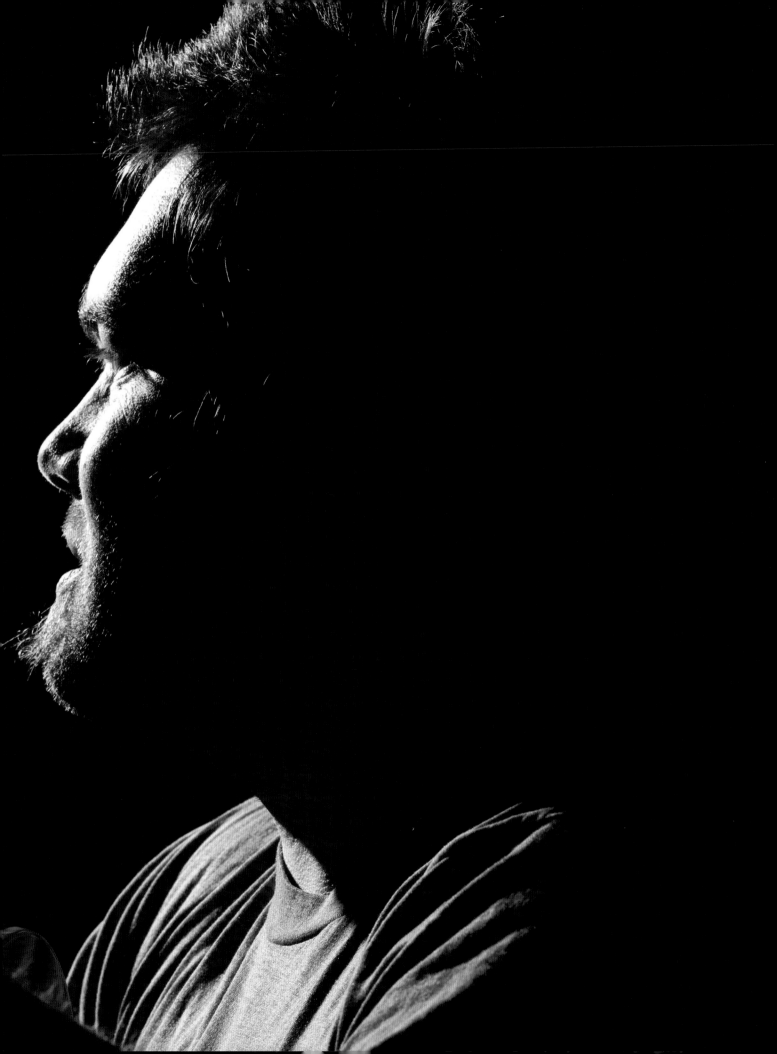

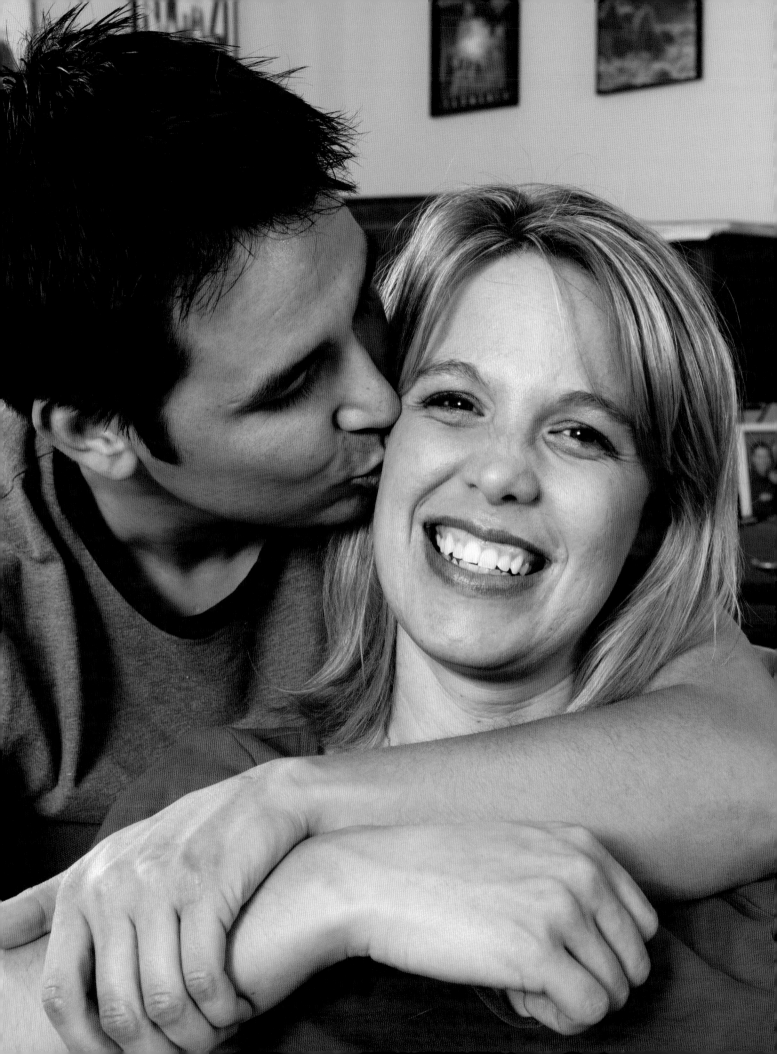

Kim Linz

Assistant Principal, Math Coach
Age at diagnosis, 28
Adrenal cancer, 2000

KIM: I was a vegetarian, training for a triathlon, and thought I was pretty healthy. And yet, while training, I had put on thirty pounds in three months. Soon after my diagnosis, they removed a tumor the size of a grapefruit. I was put on a mixture of two chemotherapy drugs plus two oral chemo drugs for six three-week cycles. Watching that orange fluid go into my portacath, I had to believe the poison would make me better. I have been on oral chemotherapy for fourteen years now and have been told I always will be. There is a very low chance of survival for this cancer, but I always knew I was going to survive. One doctor told me that I was a spoiled brat about my cancer; I would not give up.

Dave and I were not yet married. I feel so lucky that he stayed. He's a real gift, and I credit my survival to his staying right here with me. It's amazing what he did for me at age twenty-eight. Dave and our dog, Mattie, never left my side. I can't emphasize how important it was to have her here as well. Mattie's inexplicable sense of what was going on was a constant reassurance to me. I call her the little person in the fur coat.

Dave thinks it's harder for the person with cancer, but we disagree on that. I can judge what I can and cannot do, but he can't, so he felt like he had no control. Also, he didn't feel that it was fair to talk about his resentments and having to do everything around the house.

DAVE, KIM'S HUSBAND: I was often angry, but I didn't know what to do with it. It seemed preposterous to be angry with the person with cancer. What could possibly be more insensitive than that? I worried about what would happen to me if I had to go on without her, but I couldn't bring that up because it seemed pessimistic. I learned that we had to talk about everything.

KIM: There were times when I also felt like I had no control. Now something else was running my life. One of the biggest lessons for me has been to learn what I can and cannot control. Sometimes I have to let go. That's why I carry the serenity prayer in my purse.

I have developed a new sense of normal. I've forgotten what the old normal feels like. So many things are more valuable to me, such as my love for my family. I had to give up having children as a result of this illness, so my family back home is very important.

And my time is valuable. I used to be a yes person; now I protect my time and my space. I no longer need to be the star. I'm a stronger person, and I have become someone that people can lean on. I almost don't recognize this person.

We went from being two individuals to being a team, a very brave team. If we can do this, what can't we do?

I never thought it was possible to get back some of what I lost twelve years ago. I am now able to handle a stressful, demanding job as an elementary school principal and am training to do a half marathon—my first since right before my diagnosis. Cancer no longer is what defines me. Instead, my roles as a wife, aunt, daughter, sister, and friend are my defining roles. I am also far more willing to share my experience to help others from a position of strength and inspiration.

DAVE: Our relationship really changed. We've become closer and we communicate better. We went quickly from being a young couple to an older, wiser couple. But that wisdom is almost wasted, because no one our age understands, even if we try to describe it. This kind of wisdom has to be learned on your own.

My biggest lesson has been that everything is temporary. There is an illusion that life goes on forever. The only guarantee is what I have right now.

KIM: And what we have is a unique bond, thanks to cancer. We're old souls now. We went from being two individuals to being a team, a very brave team. If we can do this, what can't we do?

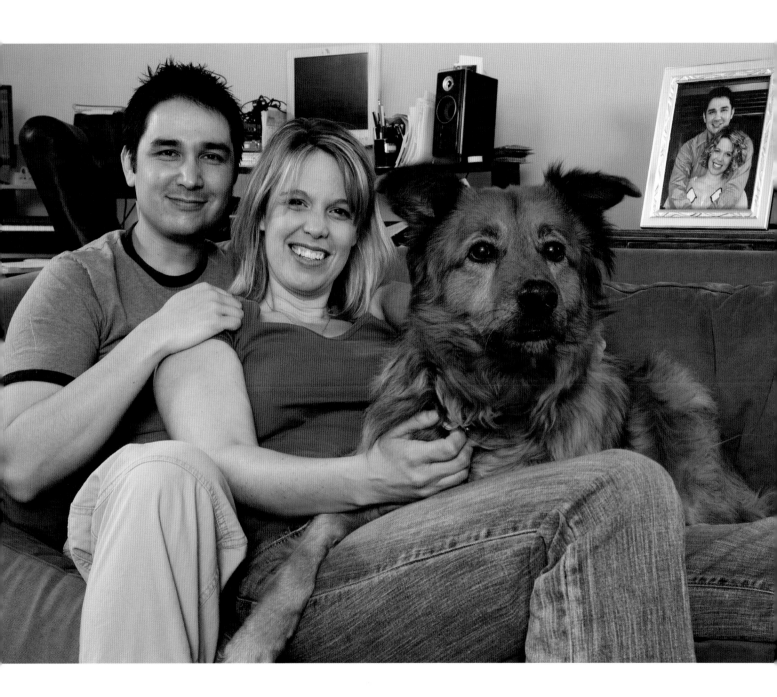

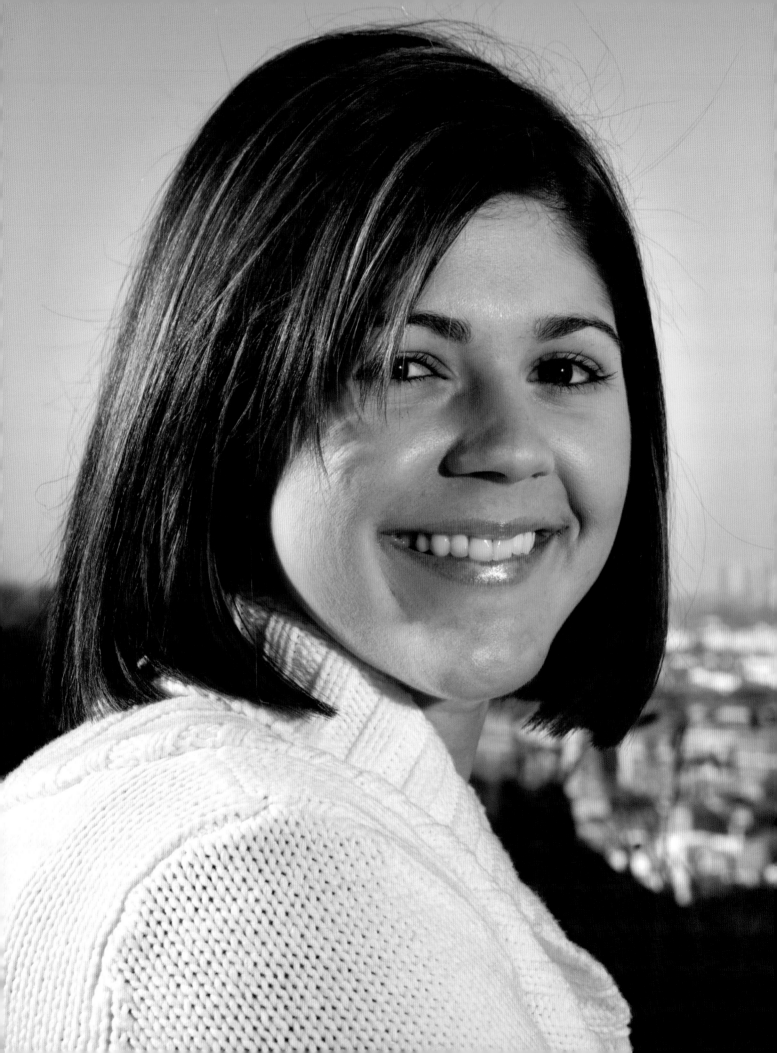

Kristina Alarcon

Teacher
Age at diagnosis, 5
Acute lymphoblastic leukemia (ALL), 1991

I was five years old. I spent a lot of time sick in the hospital and then had two years of chemotherapy. The thing I most remember, though, was being too sick to go to Disneyland while everyone else went.

When you're a child, you don't have a perception of death. You only know you're sick. Chemo to me meant something good afterward. If another kid in the hospital didn't survive, I couldn't understand what that meant.

Cancer is always there in my mind. It informs how I live my life. I was given the opportunity to live, unlike a lot of others. That is a responsibility; I need to get out there and live life to the fullest and do things. There isn't much that I won't try. I'd rather try, try really hard, and not succeed, than never try at all.

Because of cancer, I am much more sensitive as a teacher. Kids will often mask what is going on at home. They just need someone to talk to, someone who won't judge.

You never know who has been affected by cancer. It could be the person standing next to you or passing you on the street. I think about that a lot.

I had a college scholarship from the American Cancer Society, which required a number of hours of community service. The group holds a yearly luncheon for all the recipients, and it is amazing to see all these kids who are doing so much to help the world. One year I was asked to be the guest speaker.

I would never want to go back and erase cancer from my life. Absolutely not. It's part of my identity. Because cancer has been in my past, it is also a huge part of where I am going. It affects how I want to treat everyone around me. In the end, cancer became a positive experience because it affects how I make an impact on the world.

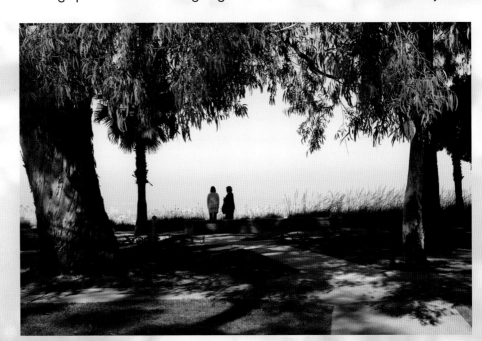

I'd rather try, try really hard, and not succeed, than never try at all.

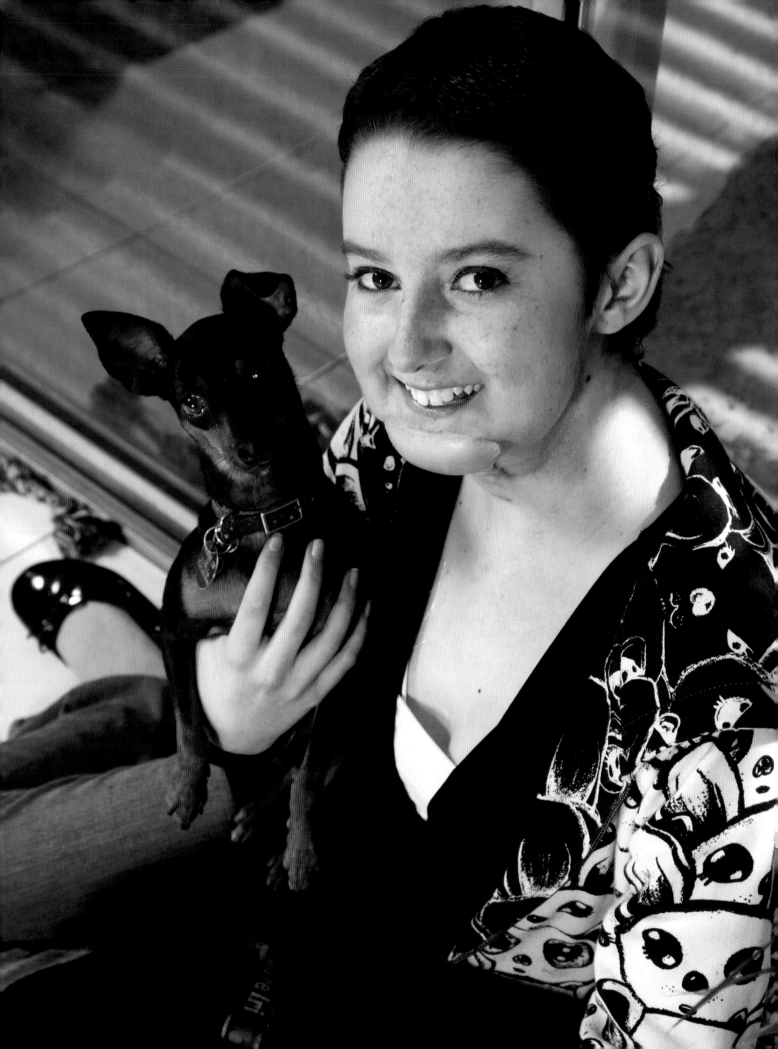

Kylie Williams

Age at diagnosis, 14
Myofibroblastic sarcoma, 2008

*L*ISA, KYLIE'S MOM: Her cancer is so rare that they didn't know what it was. There were only eight documented cases of it in the world. After three months of chemotherapy, she developed two more tumors, so she had to have surgery to remove her entire lower jaw. They used a titanium plate and a piece of her leg to reconstruct the outside of her mouth and used tissue from her arm for the inside.

We were all in shock at first, but we didn't want to waste time on that. We just started focusing on getting the problem solved. We knew it was going to be a long road ahead, and we've all remained strong through it. There was never any "Why us?" We took the attitude that it is what it is, so let's deal with the problem.

KYLIE: There are two choices. You do or you die, so we just "did." At first I was angry and wanted to know what I did to cause it, but then I just went with the flow because I didn't have a choice. My theme has become "Kick butt daily."

My theme has become "Kick butt daily."

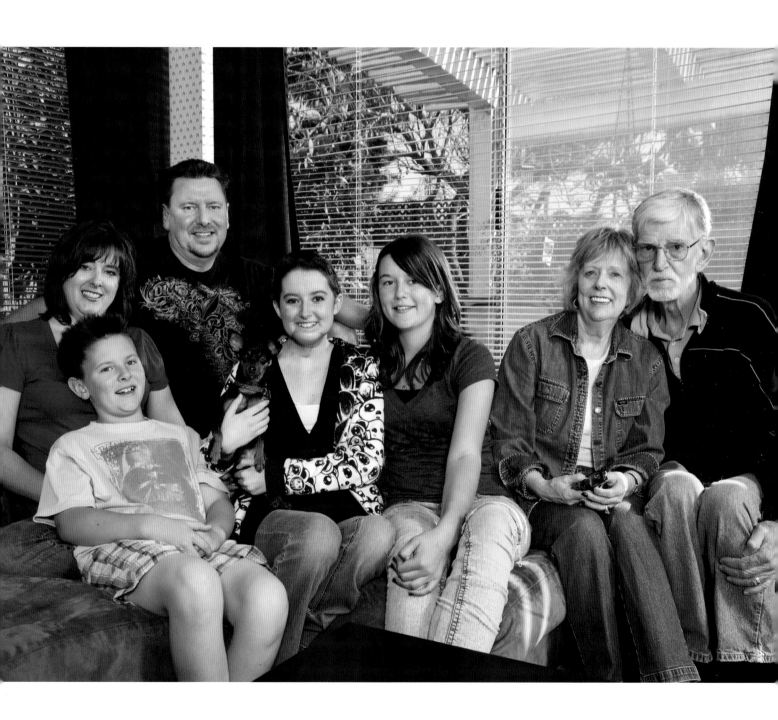

In many ways, this has helped our family. We spend a lot more time together because now we see how fast it can all be taken away.

Lisa: It has made our three kids closer. Of course there has been a little jealousy, but there is now a lot more compassion and understanding. The whole process has also made Heath and me more patient. The kids might not agree with that, but we definitely are.

Cancer can often cause divorce because of exhaustion and high frustration levels. We had to learn to not take it out on each other. In the long run, it has made our love much stronger. Because of spending all those months dealing with something so serious, everything is put in perspective. Now that we are beginning to return to normal, Heath and I take more time for each other. Even if it's just running to the store, we do it together.

Heath, Kylie's dad: I often have to leave for work at 5:00 a.m., and I don't get home until late. This has completely changed my perspective about the time I have with my family. We also now feel that anyone who has had cancer, especially children, is part of our extended family. It is a parent's worst nightmare, so we want to help other families whenever we can.

Lisa: Paying it forward is an absolute necessity. We have to help others, because too many people have been too good to us.

> *It is a parent's worst nightmare, so we want to help other families whenever we can.*

Having cancer in the family is devastating. On the other side, there are positives. One is that Kylie and I are so much closer. How many mothers with a fourteen-year-old teenager can say that?

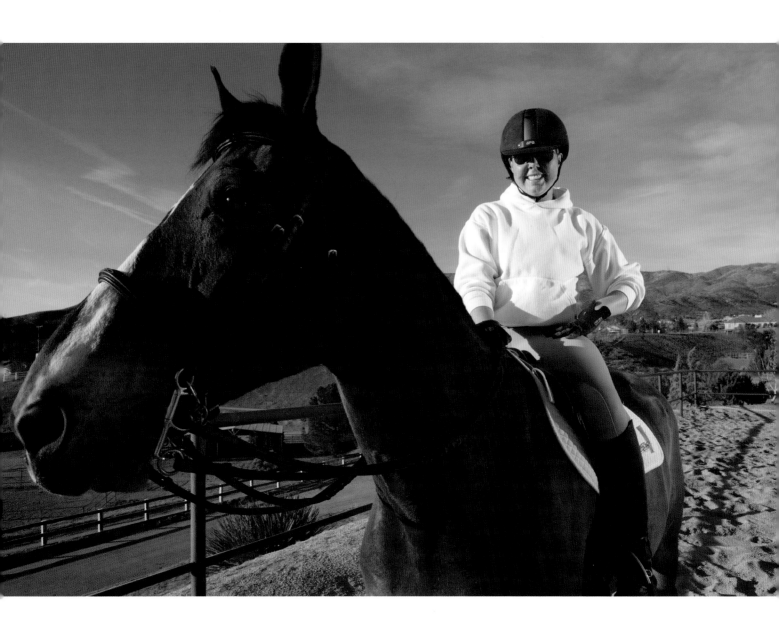

Lacy Stormes

Student, California State, Northridge
Age at diagnosis, 22
Non-Hodgkin's lymphoma, stage 3, 2008
Recurrence, 2009

*L*ACY: The cancer had gone from my circulatory system into my central nervous system and spread to my brain and my lungs. It was so severe they had to induce a coma for two weeks. The first thing I said to the doctor was, "When can I get home, ride horses again, and kick this thing in the butt?" I've always been strong and a natural competitor, and never backed down from a fight. Not long after that, I realized it's not quite as easy being strong when you're bald.

I usually push ahead and take on too much instead of playing it safe. Cancer has made me listen to that other side. It tells me to make good decisions, to do the mature thing.

Before this, I was egotistical. Now I feel humbled and vulnerable. I couldn't do everything for myself, so I had to rely on others. I changed emotionally. I am much more social and take my connections with other cancer patients very seriously. Those connections are more precious than any I had known before, and they are instantaneous and strong. My whole being seems driven to help others, rather than just focusing on me. I like the post-cancer Lacy better.

CANDICE, LACY'S MOM: She is more determined than ever before. This has broadened her to try new things; she seems to have no boundaries. Very little scares her now. She'll say to people, "I've been through cancer; what's your story?" And everyone is so attracted to that strength and courage. When she left the ICU, the doctors and nurses gave her a standing ovation.

"I've been through cancer; what's your story?"

LACY: In 2009 I found out that my cancer had returned. I had to do chemo again, and then had a stem cell transplant in 2010. I headed right to the salon to get my hair cut into a Mohawk before I had to shave it again. I am now in remission and am healthy and have returned to a full-time competition schedule with the horses.

I was Miss California in 2007, so I've been to the top and I've been to the bottom. Most people my age don't understand the things I have had to learn. Since I was already intimidating to guys my age, I'm hoping I can find someone just as strong. The men in my life have only been able to take in so much information before it's too deep for them. Then they don't want to deal with it anymore.

Sometimes I feel like I'm the only rebel left, like the song that says, "I'm the only John Wayne left in this town." But at least I'm a rebel *with* a cause.

Larry Neinstein, MD

Physician, Professor and Director of Engemann Student Health,
University of Southern California
Age at first diagnosis, 21
Metastatic melanoma, 1974
Multiple myeloma, 2005
Multiple myeloma recurrence, 2010

I was twenty-one years old. As I woke up from surgery, my wife, Debbie, my mother, and my mother-in-law were crying. I knew it couldn't be good. The melanoma had metastasized into my lymph nodes, so I had to have a second surgery for a radical removal of the other lymph nodes. As I watched them scan my body for an evaluation, each click became a click toward life or death.

There was a 5 percent chance or less that I would make it five years. My question to myself was, *Do I get an internship at a hospital, or do I go to Tahiti and sit on the beach?* I ended up doing both. I became an intern and resident at Cedars Sinai Hospital working with teens, and I traveled all over Europe.

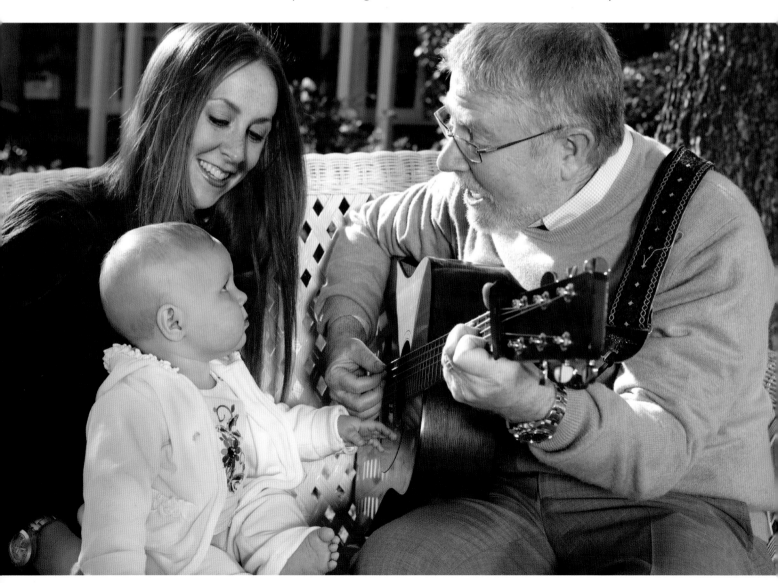

Since then, I have traveled all over the world but have continued to be highly active in my professional career. I developed an amazing reaffirmation of life and an attitude of hope. I have shared that with many other survivors and have spoken to many groups.

Then in 2005 I had a tremendous pain in my back that wouldn't get better. I discovered I had multiple myeloma. I have continued to survive due to a successful bone marrow transplant and very difficult treatments. I refer to my ongoing chemotherapy as "appetizer chemo, main course chemo, dessert chemo, and triple high-dose atomic blasts." In spite of it, I have remained active, filled with family, work, hikes, music, trips abroad, and speaking engagements. I refuse to give in.

I am currently not in remission, and my levels still go up and down, but my quality of life is good. I have less of the disease than a few years ago. It constantly reaffirms the fragility of life, which keeps me from under-appreciating the moments that seem to go in slow motion. They feel like hours, because they are so valuable. As George Carlin said, "It's not the number of breaths you take. It's the moments that take your breath away."

The soul, I think, is only a flickering light when we are born. It gains and grows in strength, meaning, and depth throughout our lives, through our families, friends, colleagues, and through profound moments of things like music and dance. At the same time, our soul is partially emptying itself to our children and everyone we touch.

I had an "aha!" moment as I was staring into my one-month-old granddaughter's eyes, and she was staring back with a combination of emptiness and fullness, of love and yearning, waiting for her soul to have a chance at so much to come. I realized at that moment that my soul is in so many places and people, and continues to flourish in their lives.

Do I get an internship at a hospital, or do I go to Tahiti and sit on the beach?

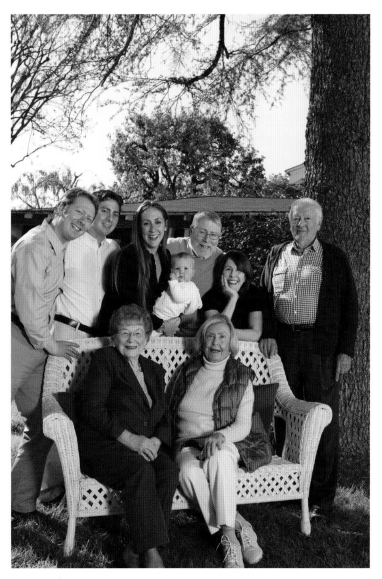

Back row (left to right): Aaron Neinstein (our son), David Neinstein (our son), Yael Afriat, our daughter, and her daughter Bella], Larry Neinstein; Debbie Neinstein, my wife, married forty years in 2012 and married a little over one year after my diagnosis of cancer, and Ben Barak (debbie's father).
Bottom row: Shirley Neinstein, my mother, and Roz Barak, debbie's mother.

141

Noga Sherman (mother)

Docent Coordinator at the Skirball Museum
Age at diagnosis, 43
Non-Hodgkin's lymphoma, stage 4, 1992
Recurrence, 1994
Second recurrence, 1997

Lauren Sherman Becker (daughter)

Nurse-Practitioner
Age at diagnosis, 24
Hodgkin's lymphoma, stage 3, 2003
Recurrence, 2009

NOGA: It was a tough year for our family. My father-in-law died in July, my mother died in November, and my mother-in-law died the next July, on the day I was diagnosed. When I walked into the office of my husband, a physician, I saw his head on his desk; he had just received the news of his mother. Then we went downstairs to find out I had cancer.

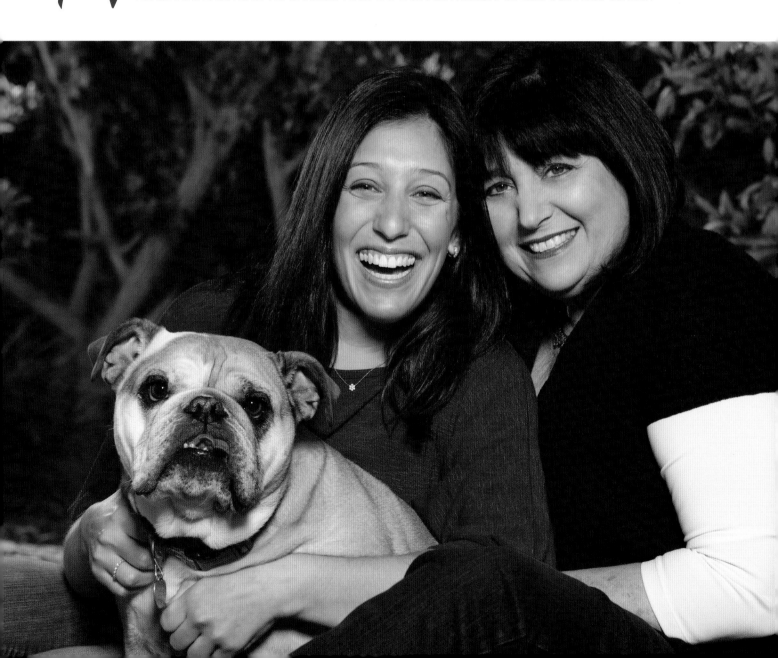

The treatments were difficult. After five years and two recurrences, I participated in a clinical trial at Stanford. This time I was determined to take control and get over it. When they gave me chemo, I said, "May I have some more please?" My husband says that I amazed him. I couldn't let it change my life because I still had to be a mom.

> ## I couldn't let it change my life because I still had to be a mom.

As difficult as it was, none of it was as difficult as when Lauren got sick.

LAUREN: And it was the opposite for me. It was harder for me when Mom was sick.

I was working in San Francisco and flying back and forth to LA every week for my consulting job. I was also training for a race and not getting as much rest as I needed. When I complained about being tired, my mother told me to slow down.

My first reaction when I was diagnosed was a sense of guilt. Our family had already been through so much. Now everything had to revolve around me.

It surprised me how I started treating everyone. I'm normally pretty sweet, compassionate, and open, but I started pushing people away. I knew I wasn't going to die, but everyone's calls and care packages made me feel that way. On the night of my diagnosis, my parents had all their friends over, and it felt like a funeral. The nicest thing was just having my brother come sit and watch TV with me.

NOGA: All I wanted to do was make Lauren feel better. When I took her to a pet store, she saw a puppy that made her laugh. We bought her and named her Emma, which means nurse or healer.

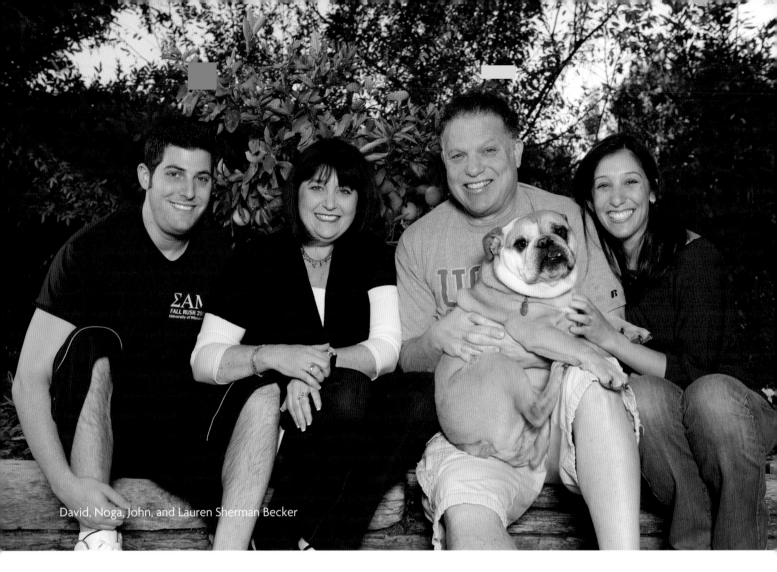

David, Noga, John, and Lauren Sherman Becker

LAUREN: Emma really gave me a sense of purpose while I was sick. When I was with her, I didn't have to talk.

I went back to work, but it didn't feel the same. I was different, and I wasn't comfortable. I felt like I could be doing so much more, but I didn't know what. A friend of mine, who told me that I am smart and have a gift, lit a fire under me when he said, "Just do it." Since I wanted to help patients and their families, I moved to New York City and completed my nursing and nurse-practitioner degrees at Columbia University.

> *I felt like I could be doing so much more . . .*

In 2008, I ran a marathon benefitting the Leukemia and Lymphoma Society. I wanted to prove to myself that I was healthy. While I was running the twenty-six miles, I took in deep breaths and appreciated the ability to do what I was doing. It was a powerful feeling.

From now on, career will never be number one. I will always put my family and friends first. In the long run, this has made our family stronger. When I tell other people about us, they are in awe. I just feel like it's normal and we're like any other family.

NOGA: I have been cancer-free since 1999. I continue to enjoy my good health by spending time with my friends and family (and Emma) as well as working as the docent coordinator at the Skirball Museum.

I still, however, have this little person in the back of my brain asking, *Are we done now in our family? Is this over?*

LAUREN: A week after completing my nurse practitioner program at Columbia University and three weeks before my wedding, I was diagnosed with a recurrence of my Hodgkin's lymphoma. After our wedding, I had more chemo and then an autologous stem cell transplant at City of Hope Hospital in May 2010. I have been in remission since my transplant. My loving husband and I cherish my good health every day. In June 2011 I started my career as a nurse practitioner with a prostate oncology practice in Los Angeles, where I can give back to the cancer community.

I have to add the mention of a miracle. In preparation for my stem cell transplant, I harvested several months' worth of eggs so that I could later have children. Those eggs, it turns out, did not work either in me or in a surrogate. Then in October 2013, I found out that, against all odds, I had become pregnant. We now are proud parents of a beautiful baby girl.

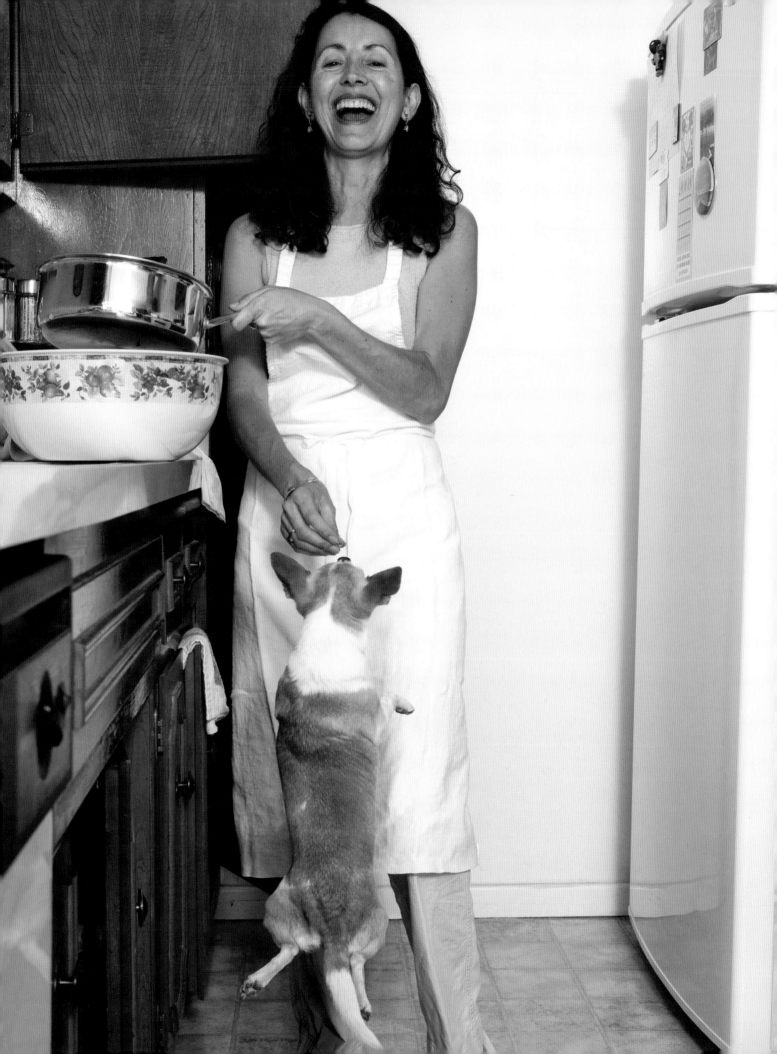

Lilly Padilla

Certified Health Coach—Holistic Nutrition
Age at diagnosis, 40
Ovarian cancer, 2003

*I*t was a time I will never forget. I changed both my work life and my romantic life at the same time. I was under a lot of stress and too busy to pay attention to my body symptoms, but I knew something was wrong.

Doctors kept telling me I was fine, but I argued and convinced them to order an ultrasound. They found a lump in one of the ovaries. When I woke up from surgery, I saw my mother crying and I knew it was cancer. From that day on, my life changed completely.

Both of my parents are very strong people. They taught me that obstacles in life are going to happen, but those obstacles are there to learn from and jump over. My whole life my father would say, "You can do it. Just jump."

I almost felt like I could not survive. But my mother and my sister were strong for me. Many of my relatives came and called me constantly, from Colombia and other countries, to support me. They asked me daily, "Today are you going to get up and learn something? Or are you going to stay in bed?"

I began to fight. I went to a psychologist to find out about caring for my mind and emotions. I also realized that I had not been taking care of my body. I began educating myself to better understand what happened to my health. I wanted to bring myself back into balance and help others do the same. I took nutrition and cooking classes and started my journey with holistic nutrition.

Through learning, I started "cleaning" my heart, my emotions, and my body. It's hard to articulate all the changes, but I completely reprogrammed myself. In the beginning, the changes were just for myself, to get healthy. Then I fell in love with holistic nutrition and went back to school to have formal training. One day I realized—this is a good thing. Without cancer, I would never have taken a look at these things and never have changed my career into something meaningful.

The best thing we can do is to be an inspiration for other people. I love helping and teaching patients and clients all the things they can do to improve their health, how to eat well, have less stress, and how to keep a balanced lifestyle.

I went from a bad experience and feeling depressed to having a wonderful life, finding my purpose, and being a much stronger person. I see the better things in life instead of worrying about the little things. I know that the way I think determines how life will unfold. If I think with a good emotion, my life will be good. And it is.

I know that the way I think determines how life will unfold. If I think with a good emotion, my life will be good. And it is.

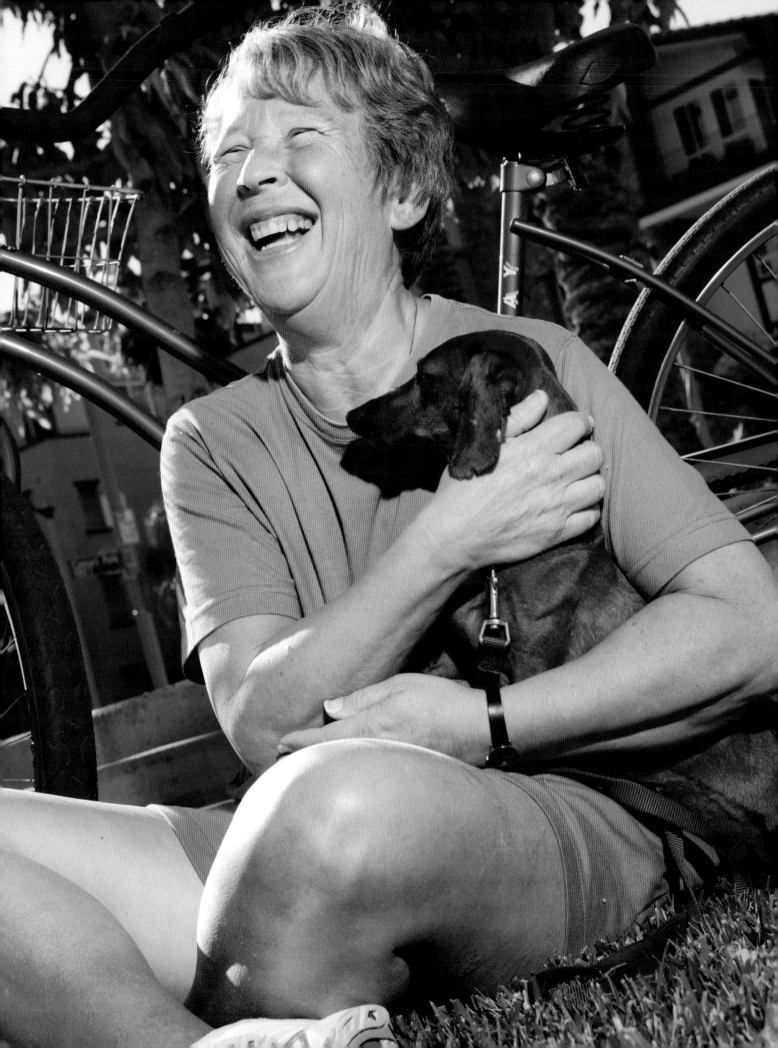

Loene Trubkin

Attorney
Age at first diagnosis, 34
Breast cancer, 1976
Fallopian tube cancer, 2006

The first time I had cancer, I was thirty-four years old. After surgery and eleven months of chemo, I bounced right back. After thirty years go by, you assume the cancer is pretty much gone.

I had just made reservations for a kayaking trip in Antarctica, a gift to myself for finishing law school and passing the bar exam. Two weeks later I was diagnosed with fallopian tube cancer. I had to postpone the trip, but the promise that one day I would kayak with the penguins kept me going through my three surgeries, chemo, and months of fatigue. The next January I was on a forty-eight-passenger Russian expedition, kayaking twice a day. It was fantastic.

I had promised myself that I would never do chemo a second time, but I found a therapist who taught me self-hypnosis and visualization. I felt like I armed myself with enough tools to have control over it. I visualized the courageous little huskies from the movie *Eight Below* seeking out and killing the cancer cells in my abdomen.

There was a point after my first cancer when I knew life was much more meaningful—I could have lost the battle. My mother and two of her sisters did lose theirs. Gradually that feeling went away and I started taking everything for granted again. I lived my life being the person who did all the planning and making sure every detail got done, as if I could control the future.

Now I am living my life much more in the now than I ever have. All we have is today. This is my life . . . today. If I hadn't gotten the second diagnosis, I know I would be a workaholic, forgetting about good friends, good food, and all the little pleasures. I remain convinced that those of us who are able to live in the present have happier and more fulfilling lives—so I keep trying to stay there.

> *. . . many of us who fight this disease find there are positives in it.*

Because so many in my family died, I held a belief that is common in the popular culture: cancer equals death. Cancer does not have to set you apart from the rest of the world. Instead, many of us who fight this disease find there are positives in it.

I now get to volunteer as an advocate for children in foster care and for low-income families with legal problems. I recently adopted a little red dachshund named Heidi. My house may never be clean again, but I don't care. Life is good.

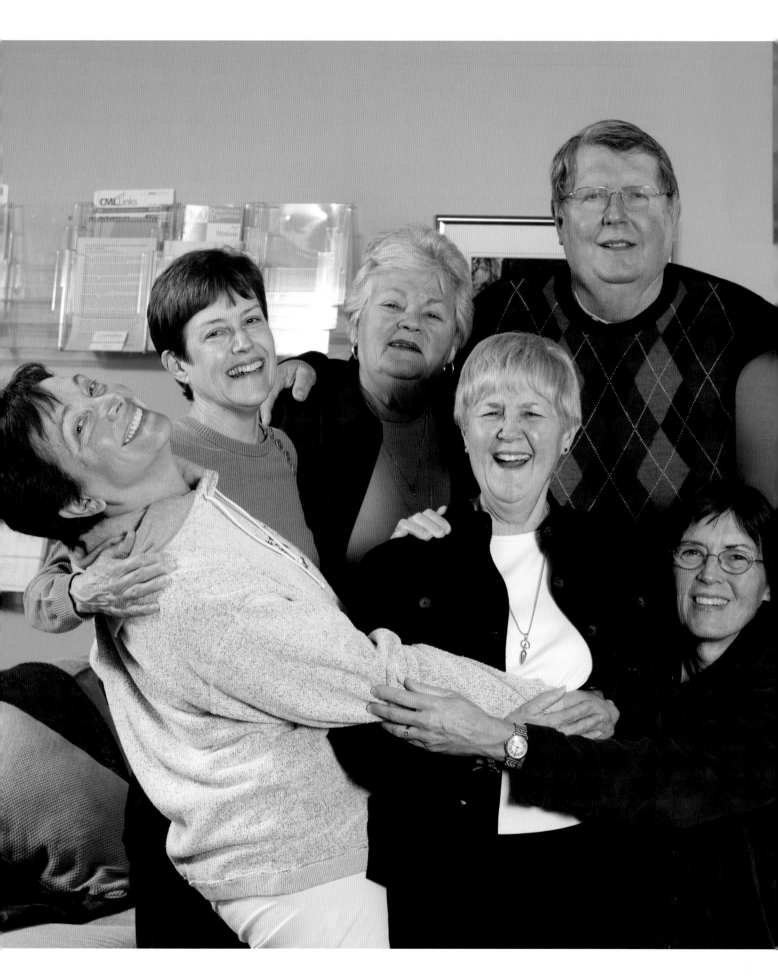

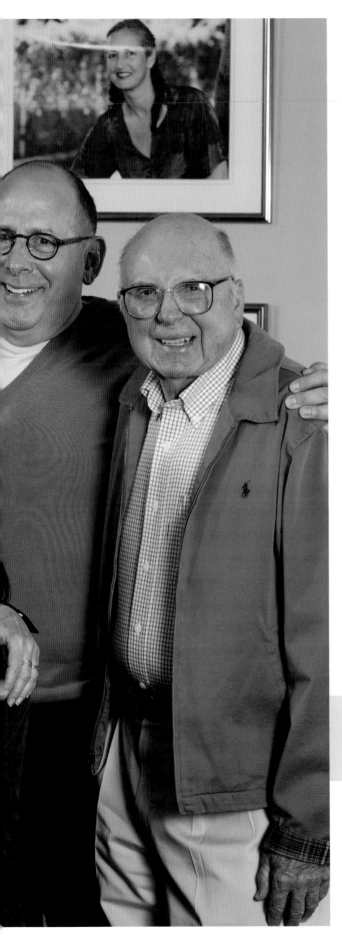

Phil Fisher

As told by his wife, Lola Fisher
Age at diagnosis, 27
Kidney cancer, 1958
Recurrence, 1979
Died, 1984

*M*y husband, Phil, was diagnosed when he was just twenty-seven years old. After treatment he remained healthy for twenty-nine years. We became so much closer. We wouldn't let mundane worries get to us.

In 1979 Phil was diagnosed with a recurrence that had metastasized to his liver. I will never forget when the doctor told us that there was nothing more to be done. He said Phil had three to six months, but we remained optimistic. Phil said he had regained his health once before, and he could do it again. From then on he did nothing but alternative treatments. Like many others, he defied the odds and lived five more years. In 1984 I finished school and became a licensed psychotherapist. Phil was there for my graduation.

When I lead cancer therapy groups, I tell them that cancer creates a new normal. It affects everyone in the family, oftentimes putting a strain on finances or creating stress because of changing roles. It also hampers normal, comfortable daily activities. Once you or a loved one has cancer, life is never the same. It is not necessarily better or worse, but it is never the same.

Like many others, he defied the odds . . .

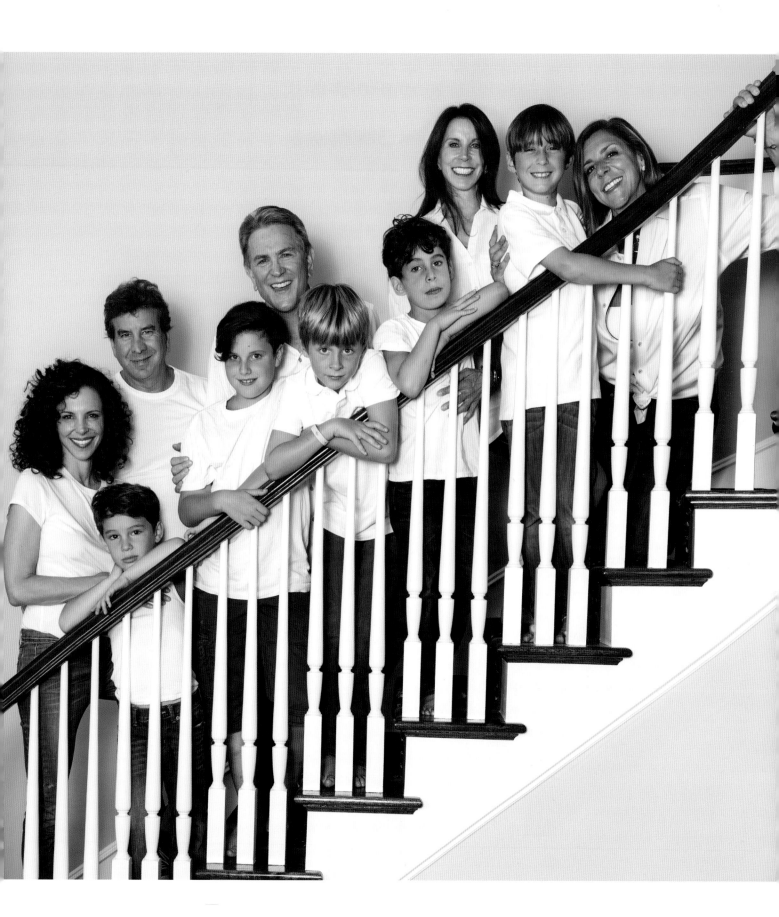

Lon Morton

Financial Advisor
Age at diagnosis, 58
Prostate cancer, 2003

*M*y first thought was, *Well, somebody has to get prostate cancer.*

Soon after my diagnosis, I was playing golf with a close friend who told me about robotic surgery. It intrigued me, so I researched the procedure. Several top urologists disagreed with the idea, but we are all responsible for our own destiny. I decided to go to the City of Hope Hospital for the robotic surgery. I was in the hospital on the treadmill a week later, and hitting golf balls two weeks after that. I followed this with hormone treatment and radiation. Some might think this was excessive, but eleven years "later", I feel pretty darn good.

From then on, my life took on a whole different vision. Cancer put a calendar on it. In 2006 I decided to create a "liquidity event" for my business, which I had spent a lifetime building. I sold my business, but it didn't mean retirement; quite the contrary, I continue to work today. And who knows—I might buy it back from the bank someday.

> ## Just look how fortunate I am. Today is the best time of my life.

I love what I do, which still includes working, but also includes sharing my life with five wonderful grandsons. Just look how fortunate I am. Today is the best time of my life. I try to look at every day as a tremendous opportunity. And it is. I get to squeeze the people I love. I get to tell the people at work how good they are and how much I appreciate them. This experience brought me to a point of realizing that I enjoy caring for the people around me, making their lives easier or better. If I find out that someone has just learned that he has prostate cancer, I will drop everything to talk to him. It is a pleasure and an honor to provide input and help.

Laughter is a wonderful healer. People who laugh live longer. They say that people who have a dog are expected to live seven years longer. But I'll tell you what: I'd rather pick up my grandsons than a dog, and when they say, "I love you, Poppy," it sends a love flash from my toes to my shoulders. I truly believe that having grandchildren is the greatest gift in the world. So if having one dog is worth seven years, five grandsons will keep me alive forever.

My wife is a pediatric nurse practitioner and is selfless. She has always been an inspiration to me. It's a little ironic that with this adversity came a feeling that our forty-two-year marriage has strengthened and become even better.

I think I'll easily make it to eighty . . . or why not ninety? I can tell you that most of my aches and pains are because of my age, not because I had prostate cancer.

I used to play baseball for the Angels and Indian organizations, and still hold some pretty good minor league pitching statistics. Now I have an entirely new kind of statistic. I feel very fortunate that I can turn my cancer around and help others. I was able to help the City of Hope raise $400,000 to invest in their third da Vinci machine for robotic surgery.

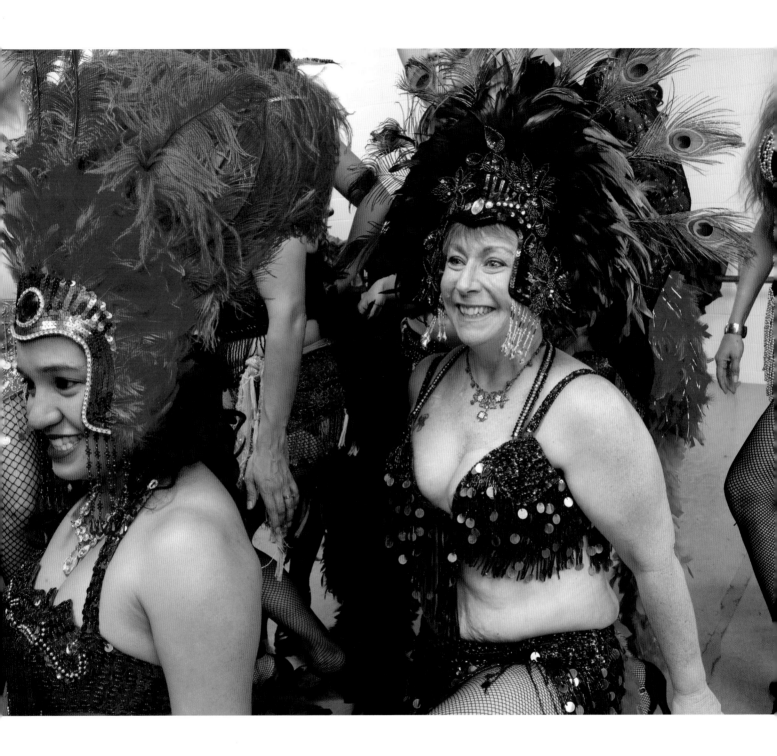

I no longer celebrate my actual birthday. My celebration is on the date of my diagnosis—my "re-birthday."

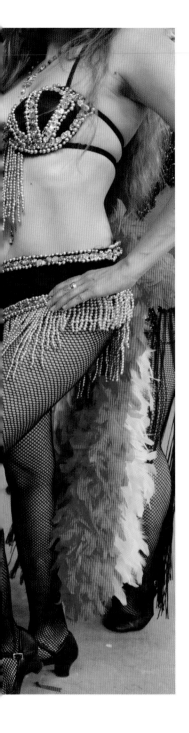

Lori Flagg | Nurse Manager
Age at diagnosis, 47
Inflammatory breast cancer, 2002

I became involved in the three-day breast cancer walk in 1999. I walked for two years and then volunteered as a medical team captain the third year. In 2002, right after my fourth walk, I noticed my breast was swollen and red. I went in for an ultrasound and had immediate surgery. Doctors told me that my prognosis was not good.

I refused to consider the option of dying. It never occurred to me. I got my family together and told them we were not going to boo-hoo. We were going to treat it and move on. I knew I was willing to spend all of my energy pushing uphill. I want to live to be a hundred and make my kids miserable.

I hated physical therapy; nurses are the worst patients. Instead, I started belly dancing. At first I looked like Lucy in the chorus line. As things progressed, I recovered almost all of the range of motion in my arms and chest, gained self-confidence, and achieved a new lust for life.

These classes make me feel feminine again. I'm the oldest in the group, but these women have become my daughters, sisters, mothers, and friends. I never would have thought I could get on stage in front of an audience, but I have gone from "I can't do this" to "I can hardly wait." Dear God, I get up on stage half naked, and now my only fear is that something might fall out. I can't believe that at this age I get to have this much fun. I took the family on a cruise to Alaska to celebrate my ten years of survival. It was *awesome*!

My life really changed. Before cancer I was doing a lot of volunteering for other people. I realized that I wanted to explore things for me and express a new personality that was coming out. The learning experience from cancer has been far greater than the price.

While I was in chemo, my daughter and I got matching tattoos: a Celtic knot made of hearts at our ankles. My husband says we are exactly alike and thick as thieves. My other tattoos are a breast cancer ribbon above my "good" breast, orchids on my back for prosperity, and koi as symbols of longevity.

Speaking of age, I no longer celebrate my actual birthday. My celebration is on the date of my diagnosis—my "re-birthday."

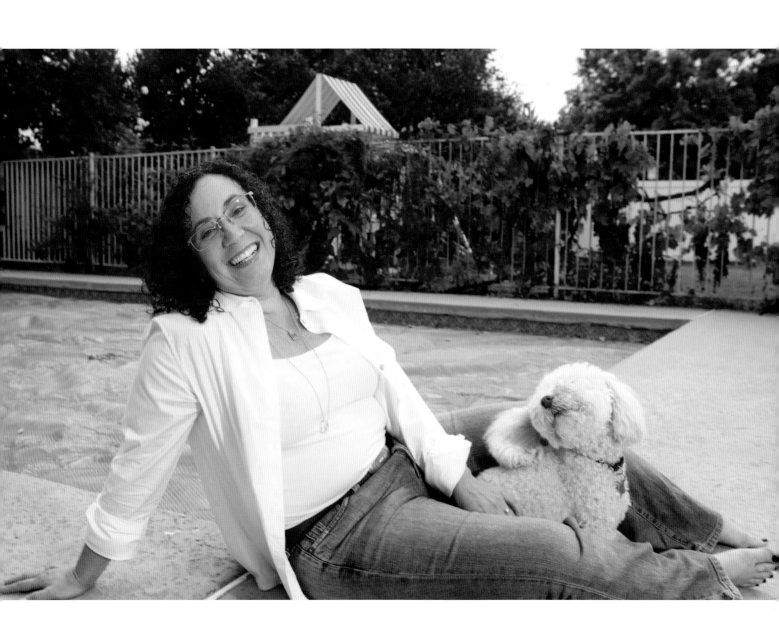

Lori Marx-Rubiner

Program Director
Age at diagnosis, 36
Breast cancer (lobular carcinoma), 2002

As soon as I got my diagnosis, my life turned upside down. I didn't know how to make decisions, where to go for the answers, or even how to ask the questions. There were intense levels of conversation about fertility and harvesting eggs and more. All of this happened at an age when I felt immortal.

One of the first challenges was explaining it to our three-year-old son. We found a book titled *The Hope Tree,* which explained cancer like a weed in a beautiful garden. We talked about surgical choices like pulling out weeds or chemotherapy as a chemical option.

Children are very aware of the energy in their home. We needed to explain that it was going to be a hard road, but we stayed very positive. I wanted to be as confident as I could for him. The main message was "You can ask us anything." And if it was too scary to come to us, he could go to any other adult he felt comfortable with.

The night I got home from my surgery, he crawled in bed with me, rubbed my arm, and said, "I'm really glad you didn't die when they pulled out the weeds."

One blessing in the Morning Prayers says that it is a miracle that our bodies work. That was the single biggest awakening of my healing. There are so many things we don't talk about: a sense of sexuality, of femininity, or a feeling of being scarred. You have to have a partner who is willing to go there with you. For us, the community also stepped up like I never would have imagined.

"Why me?" was the wrong question for me. "Why not me?" is the better question. "Why me?" keeps you stuck there. "Why not me?" puts you back into the world again. As far as I'm concerned, you've given up the battle when you ask, "Why me?"

I worried that after my treatments I would forget to bless every moment. I wanted to remember that every day I woke up was a day that I had not been promised, and that my child is the biggest blessing I have ever been given, even when he makes me mad. And I still realize that he needs more hugs and kisses than reprimands.

I wanted to remember that every day I woke up was a day that I had not been promised . . .

My husband and I are absolutely much closer now. We communicate a lot more. We make decisions together better than we ever did. We both make sure we are living based on our priorities. I have always done what I always wanted to do. I am now doing it with a fuller heart and more wisdom than I ever did before. There is also another side to me now, which is such an added blessing: the ability to help people who are cancer survivors.

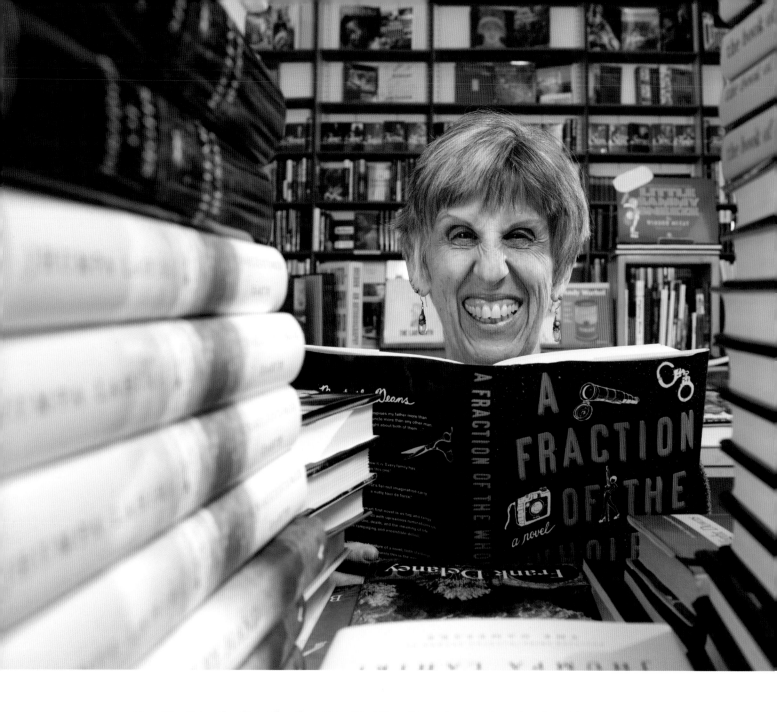

I changed my name. The old name is the person
who had cancer. Louana George does not.

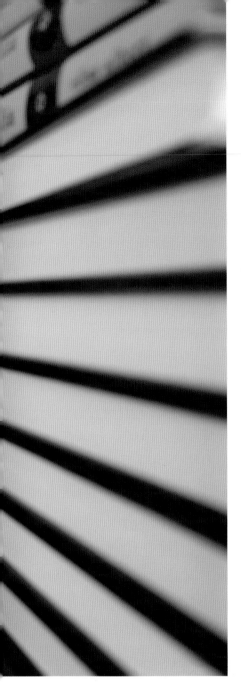

Louana George

Author, Midwife, and Nursing School Teacher
Age at diagnosis, 55
Ovarian cancer, 2005

*I*t was the year of living dangerously. I went on a medical mission for Doctors Without Borders in Liberia for five months and got malaria. I came home to recover and then went to Darfur for two months. Three months after that, I was diagnosed with ovarian cancer.

I had no health insurance, but as a self-employed health-care provider, I knew a few people to call. For the surgery, I went into debt for $30,000. For the chemotherapy, I had to resort to the county hospital, which was free, but always involved many hours of waiting for treatment.

It was a very difficult time for me. As a midwife, a huge part of my identity had to do with my uterus. Losing my hair was added humiliation. I continued to work with my patients but didn't want them to feel sorry for me because of my hair loss. They were not there to take care of me.

Now my life has completely changed. Each day has to count. Cancer might come back, or it might not, which gives me a new perspective. Life means so much more. I sold my business and my house, and I moved to Denver so I could be with my grandson. I'm now teaching in a nursing school, and I don't worry about house payments or any of that little "diddly" stuff.

I tell you what. I'm not giving up the bad stuff either. Why would I do that? I could die tomorrow, so why not enjoy today? I had a good life, I ate well, I took care of myself, and I still got cancer. So, to hell with that. Now I'm just going to be moderately good and enjoy my life. I remember an interview I heard one time with a hundred-year-old man. They asked him if he were to do his life over again, what would he do differently. He said, "I would eat more bacon."

It is now 2013 and I do not think of cancer in my life very much, if at all. I still pay attention to my body, which is what allowed me to "find" my cancer in 2005, and that suits me fine. Otherwise, I'm just like any other person living life one day at a time.

I do not want to be called a survivor. I do not want that to be my identity. I want to be clear that the cancer is not me. So I changed my name. The old name is the person who had cancer. Louana George does not.

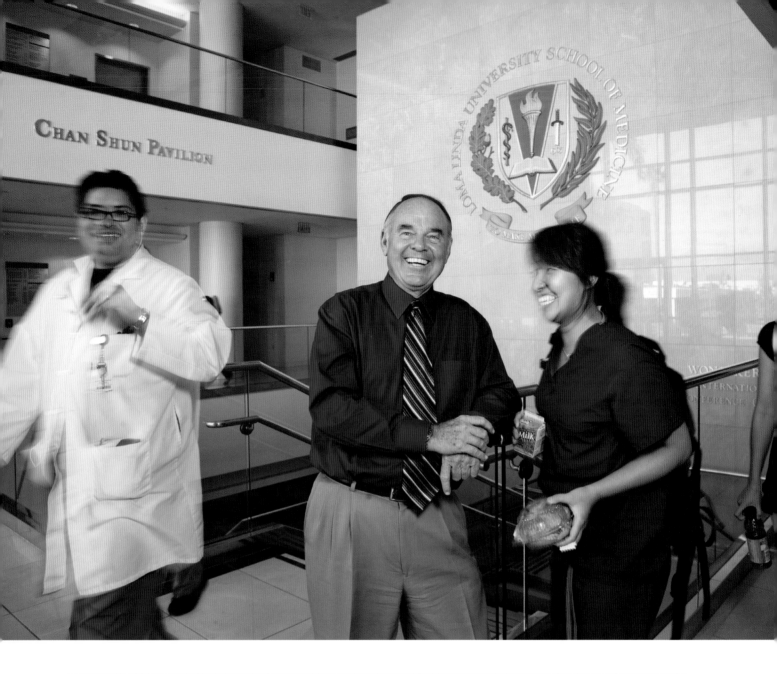

I'd like to think that on my deathbed I'll be cracking a joke.

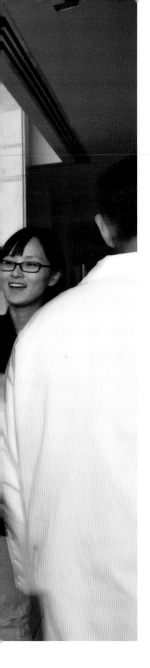

Lynn Martell

Golden Gloves Boxing Champion; Director, Special Services, Department of Radiation, Loma Linda University; Minister
Age at first diagnosis, 62
Papillary thyroid cancer, 2003
Splenic marginal zone lymphoma, 2007

I started out at a state college on a boxing scholarship. Eventually I got a Master of Divinity degree and then a doctoral degree from McCormick Theological Seminary in Chicago.

I currently produce a weekly television program for Loma Linda University called *Journey of Hope*. The primary objective of the program is to interview former patients of the medical center who have experienced some type of trauma or medical crisis. The interviewees are not only survivors; they are all *thrivers.*

I stress to our patients to stop talking about dying and instead think about how they are going to live. We all just have one day, and that's today, not tomorrow and not yesterday. Just as the psalm says, "Today is the day of the Lord. Let us be glad and rejoice in it."

Our mission as Adventists is to make man whole. We are a healing ministry: mental, physical, spiritual, and emotional. Healing is far more than just getting treatment. It is a total process. Thus, here at the Wellness Center, we offer a gym, a pool, and total health facilities. I lead an educational support group meeting for 120 people. We have professionals speak on several topics. We even take tours of restaurants to discuss nutrition.

In 1999 I was in Hawaii getting ready to climb a mountain in South America. I went for an EKG, and they saw something unusual. They shockingly referred to my angiogram as "the widow maker." One year later exactly, I went and climbed the mountain. There is life after heart surgery, just as there is after cancer.

My second diagnosis of cancer was a little different because there was no known cure for it. All of our clocks are ticking. I just hear mine ticking a little louder now. As they say, "The only thing terminal is life." As a minister, I look at things differently than most people. For the first time, I'm thinking about my own death. It helps me to recognize that there is a very real and tangible time for everyone. We can't control that, but we can choose how to live. This puts an emphasis on the knowledge that I want to live my life to the fullest.

I'd like to think that on my deathbed I'll be cracking a joke.

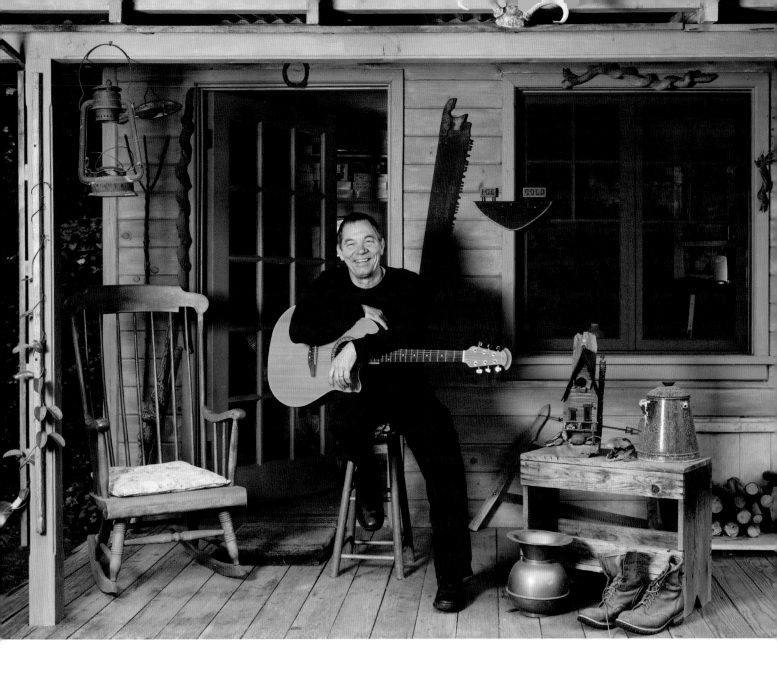

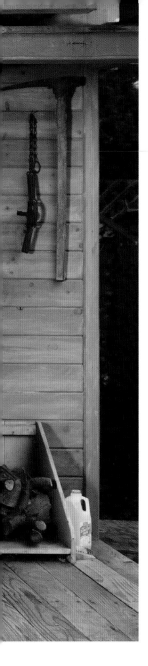

Mack Dryden

Comedian, Author
Age at first diagnosis, 34
Testicular cancer, 1988
Choroidal melanoma, 2004

The news buckled my knees and knocked the breath out of me. When the doctor told me I would go into surgery and lose a testicle, I reminded him that we were talking about one of my personal favorite organs. Over the years we'd gotten kind of attached.

I had full confidence in the medical profession to save me, so I kept it all to myself. I didn't tell anyone, including my parents or my five-year-old daughter, whom I was raising. I didn't want to burden anyone or cause them to worry about something they couldn't control. I felt that telling my parents would be like giving them the disease because they would suffer so much. When it was all over, I sent a humorous letter to everyone telling them what had happened and letting them know we had had a family triumph.

Six years later came bout number two. I became one of six in a million people to get a malignant melanoma on the back of my eyeball. I told the doctor I have no luck with my round organs. During the radiation procedure, which cost me the vision in my eye but saved my life, he told me to come up with another joke about the ordeal. I told him, "Now I'm half blind and half nuts," and got a good laugh.

After the first cancer, I felt fortunate and grateful. I appreciated life and thanked God for all my many blessings. I felt like I had been given a second life. Attitude has a lot to do with healing. It has healthful physical benefits. Why not have a good attitude and give yourself every opportunity? I got as many laughs as I could out of the whole situation.

I had always been a hard-charging, type-A person, but after cancer, I focused that on achieving things I had been putting off, like finding my soul mate and writing a book.

> It makes no sense to me not to enjoy life.

Being positive and keeping a good sense of humor will always have a positive effect; being negative and depressed will always have a negative effect. It makes no sense to me not to enjoy life. I want to laugh, to see beauty, and to leave this earth with good references: "Plays well with others." I might get a better room.

Cancer and comedy have taught me to never forget: Falling on your face is still moving forward.

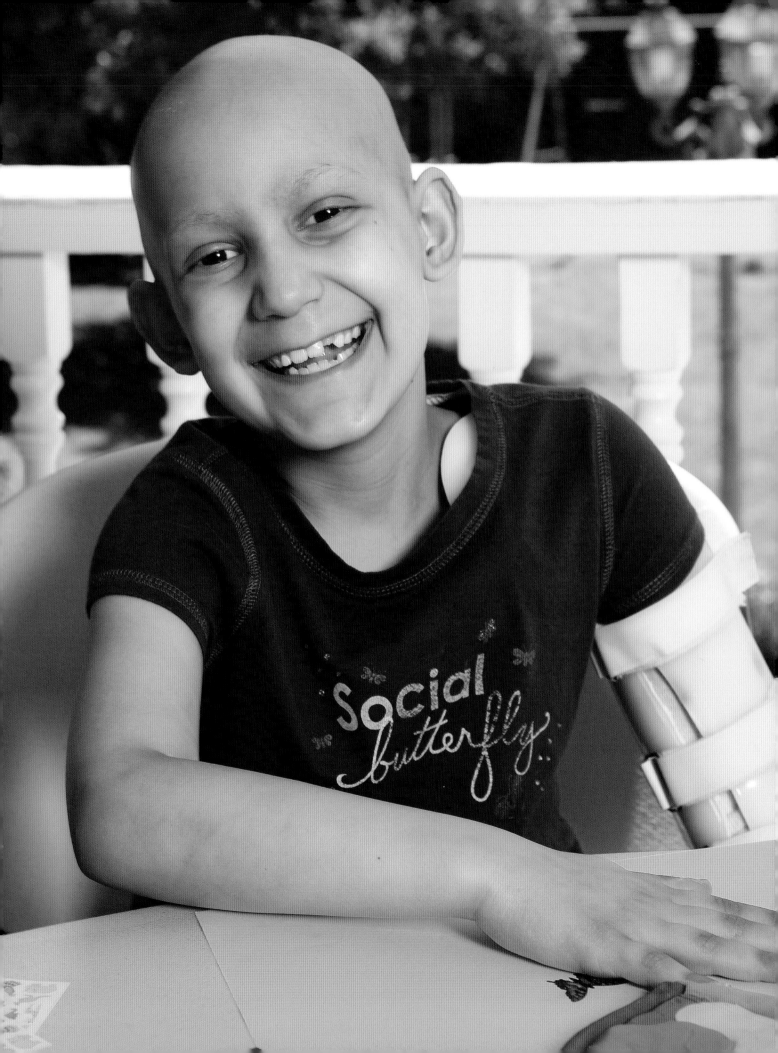

Maneh Nazarian | Age at diagnosis, 7
Bone cancer (Ewing's sarcoma), 2007

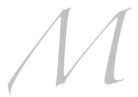 ARINE, MANEH'S MOTHER: When she was little, she loved her long hair. After we shaved her head, she looked in the mirror and said, "I may look ugly on the outside, but inside Maneh is beautiful. So don't cry, Mommy." She then started laughing and singing, "Don't you wish your girlfriend was bald like me."

EDMOND, MANEH'S FATHER: Anything we say is not enough in comparison to the amount of wisdom and courage that she passed on to us. After her fourteen-and-a-half-hour surgery to replace the bone in her arm, she was smiling and laughing. She said, "That was it?" When she woke up, she looked at me and said, "Dad, I never nagged at anyone. I smiled the whole time." I hugged her and cried.

"Don't you wish your girlfriend was bald like me."

When things like this happen, you see life in a different dimension. Spending six hours in the park with my kids is more valuable than anything else. Every moment that you hold your child is a precious moment. Before this, I was usually thinking about a bigger car or a bigger house. Now happiness is spending time with my family, tucking the kids into bed. It has changed our lives forever.

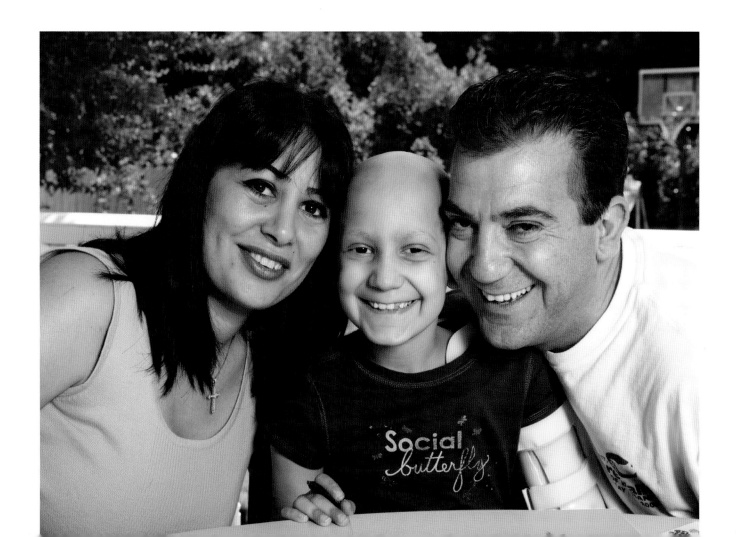

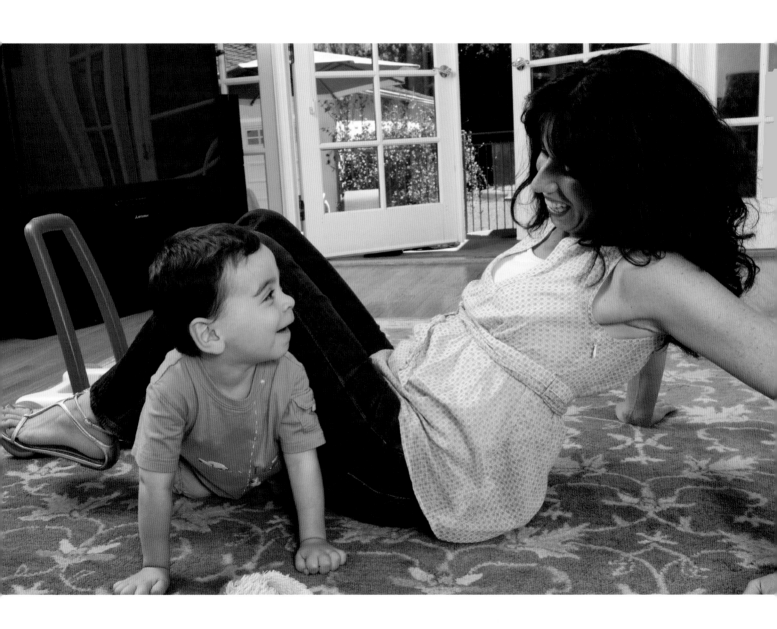

Marie Ritz

Therapist for Cancer Patients; Professor, California State, Los Angeles
Age at diagnosis, 33
Thyroid cancer, 2005

I had laryngitis, so I went to the doctor to get something simple to feel better. He felt my thyroid and sent me for an ultrasound. Then I needed a PET/CT Scan and a biopsy. Four days later, I found out that I was pregnant, which was scary because I wanted the baby more than anything. I didn't know whether to be happy or sad. I was suddenly living in a cruel irony. I was building a life inside me at the same time that something was attacking my own life.

I decided to have surgery while I was pregnant. I had to make the decision as both a mother and an expectant mother. I was afraid for my three-year-old son, Ethan, who needed me here for him. Timing the surgery was very important. I was scheduled for it when I was five months pregnant. I tell my son Dylan that he was there when Mommy had surgery. We did it together.

Dylan was born with the cord around his neck and not breathing—completely unrelated to the cancer. Thank God everything turned out all right. Now we believe that Dylan is going to be a real fighter because of how he entered the world.

Having the radiation treatment would have been extremely dangerous for Dylan. I had to do it postpartum. I was in the hospital, away from my home, and not allowed to have visitors for eleven days. It was difficult for Ethan, who is so smart. He couldn't understand why Mommy was gone so long. We put eleven granola bars in a bowl for him to eat, one every day. He knew that when they were gone, Mommy would be home. Some days he would try to eat several of them. The night I got home, he kept saying, "Look, Daddy, Mommy's here!"

As time went on, I realized that cancer *can* really change one's life for the better. It's not like anyone wants to go through it to learn this but when you find the gift, it's amazing. I had worked with cancer patients for seven years before I had it myself. Once again, another irony. I had developed a program at a cancer support center, and I knew that the post-treatment period is when all the emotions surface. That's exactly what happened to me.

> *It's not like anyone wants to go through it to learn this but when you find the gift, it's amazing.*

In the movie *Crash*, Don Cheadle's character says, "You have to crash to feel anything." That was profound for me. I needed to be hit hard to grow and heal. Having cancer is a journey that continues. There are always blood tests and medications to take. But it is a constant reminder for me to feel joy and gratitude for my health and family.

The biggest gift I have taken from having cancer is completely accepting myself and not worrying about other people's opinions of me. It is very liberating and was a tremendous shift in how I lived my life. A friend of mine put it very simply, "Oh, you mean you're telling me you're human?"

167

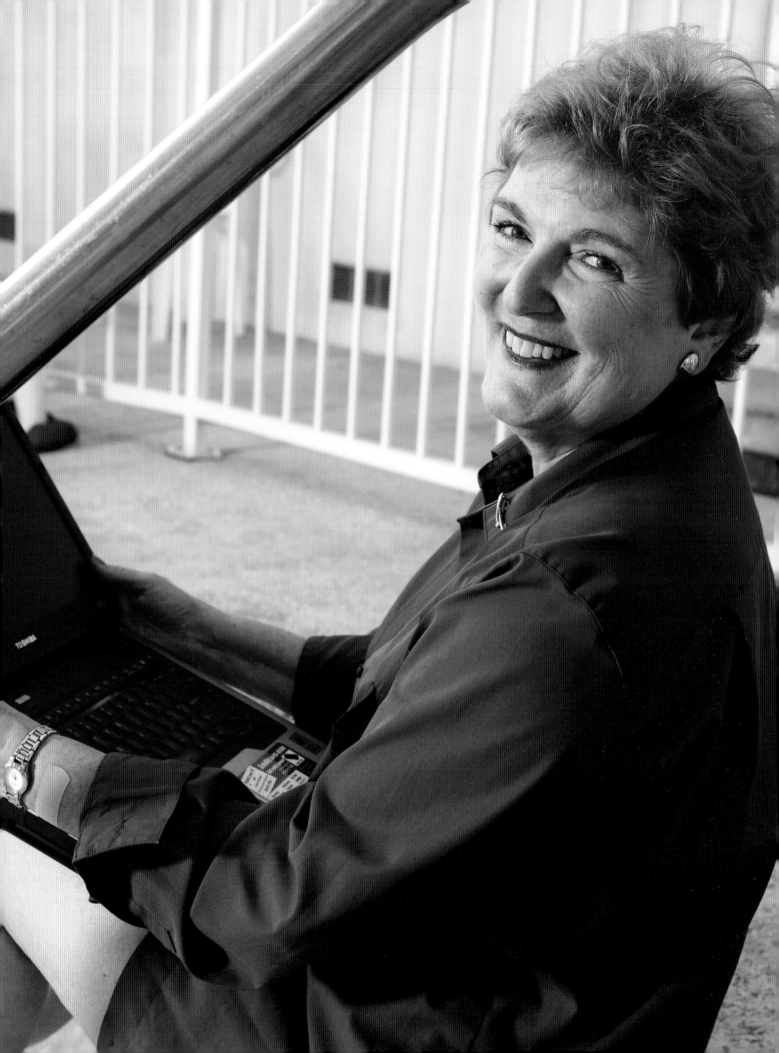

Marion Claire

Writer, Coach, Speaker
Age at diagnosis, 63
Colon cancer, 2004

My first reaction was, "Damn." Then I immediately said, "Okay, let's take care of this." Something inside me had said that it was going to be bad news, so I wasn't surprised or shocked. Dealing with it became the most important thing for me. I knew the alternative if I didn't, and yet I never once thought I was going to die from this.

I had the surgery three weeks after my diagnosis and then did six months of chemotherapy. I discovered that I had a lot more courage, and a lot more willingness to take a risk than I thought I did. It was a 180-degree flip from the rest of my life. I'm also a recovered agoraphobic, which in my mind is the fear of being anywhere you don't feel safe, physically or emotionally.

I had been a person who was never able to break the yoke of childhood. My parents loved me dearly and had the best intentions in the world, but it somehow froze me in an emotional childhood. I never knew how to think for myself and they never let me learn.

For the first time I had to be an adult. The experience gave me the courage to stand up and say, "Do it now!" I'm ready to spring myself on the world. I'm not afraid anymore. I realized that I had to be strong for myself. That's what adults do. So if you want to draw a line between childhood and adulthood, cancer is where I crossed it.

I know I'm a late bloomer, but it turns out that I'm a whole lot stronger than I ever thought I was.

Cancer for me was not a tragedy. Cancer became the gift of finding out how strong I really am. I don't know what would have happened to me if I hadn't had this gift in my life.

Cancer became the gift of finding out how strong I really am.

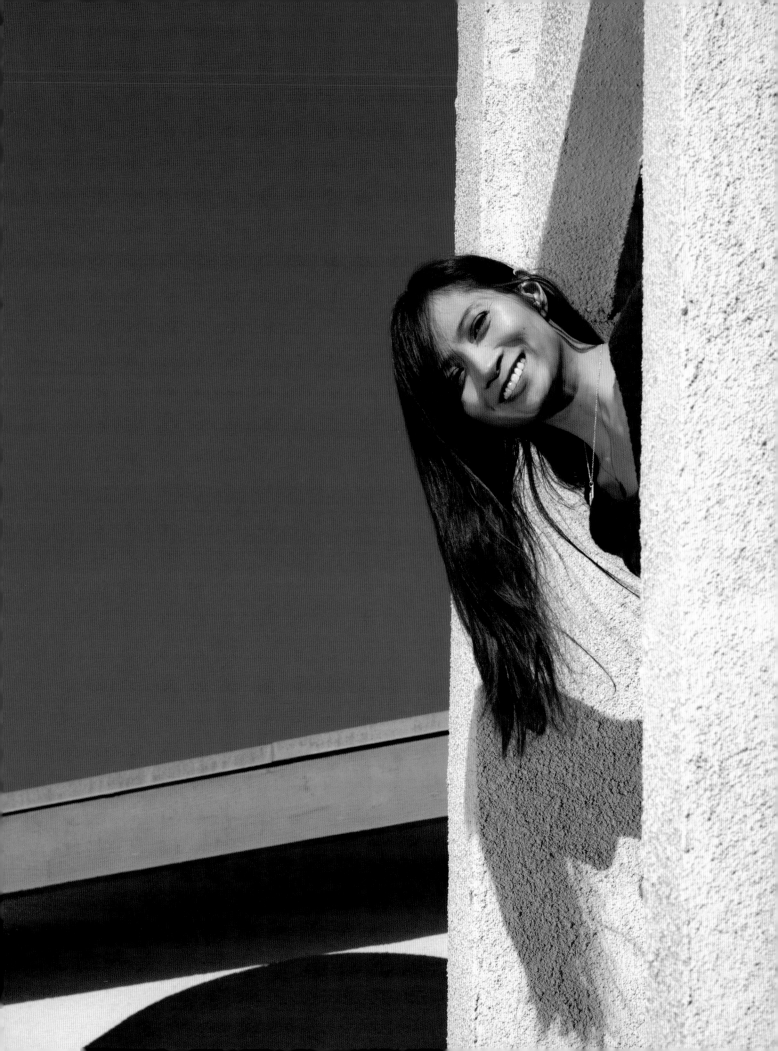

Mary Davenport

Public School Psychologist
Age at diagnosis, 31
Acinic cell carcinoma, 2008

MARY: I was married in August while in graduate school, and received my diagnosis the following May.

I was shocked and filled with a lot of anger, depression, and fear. I had to learn to shift my thinking away from the negative toward the positive. This became an opportunity for me to grow. I would call it a severe blessing, which I know is an oxymoron. I had my ass kicked, but now I know why—so I can help others.

I would call it a severe blessing, which I know is an oxymoron.

When you go through an experience like cancer, you find a lot of strength you didn't know you had. Throughout our lives, we all read about inspirational people, and then all of a sudden you have the opportunity to become one of those people. It's quite beautiful. My strength can be an inspiration to others.

In my work I deal with a lot of inner-city teenagers who live in turmoil and suffer in many different ways. They are neglected, depressed, and often suicidal. I may not be able to relate to their lives, but now I can relate to their suffering. I'm more equipped and more confident to help them.

I've learned to live a life of humble gratitude, a life of faith. Spirituality for me is about my belief that ultimately everything that happens is good for me. It's not about getting something; it's about letting go and allowing myself to grow, letting my spirit mature. I try hard to do that every day. I've also learned to love and embrace myself more. I feel grateful for the person I have become.

STEWART, MARY'S HUSBAND: This was a tough external stressor on a new marriage. I wanted to be with her through all of this. When we got married, we knew we had to roll with the punches, and this was a big one. I love her so much, but sometimes I felt excluded because she was getting support from other places. She would go through emotions she couldn't explain, and I felt at a loss. We had so much physical support during her treatments, but we had no one to help us with the emotional backlash afterward. We weren't prepared for that.

The emotional is more difficult because it's invisible.

The emotional is more difficult because it's invisible. My role was especially challenging, because I had to discern when to be her friend and rub her back, and when to say, "Now we're just in a pity party. This isn't helping you." I needed to be a coach sometimes. It was her journey, but I was certainly on the train.

Through it all, we had to mature very quickly. We both learned a lot. The experience equipped us with so much wisdom, and ultimately brought us closer together and strengthened our marriage.

Maryclare Ramirez

Age at diagnosis, 6
Soft tissue Sarcoma, otherwise
undifferentiated, 2007

E LIZABETH, MARYCLARE'S MOTHER: All the doctors just kept saying "tumor." It never clicked with me that it was cancer until they said the word *chemotherapy*. Suddenly, our world changed. Most kids wake up and go to school every day. She woke up and we went to the hospital, the clinic, or the lab.

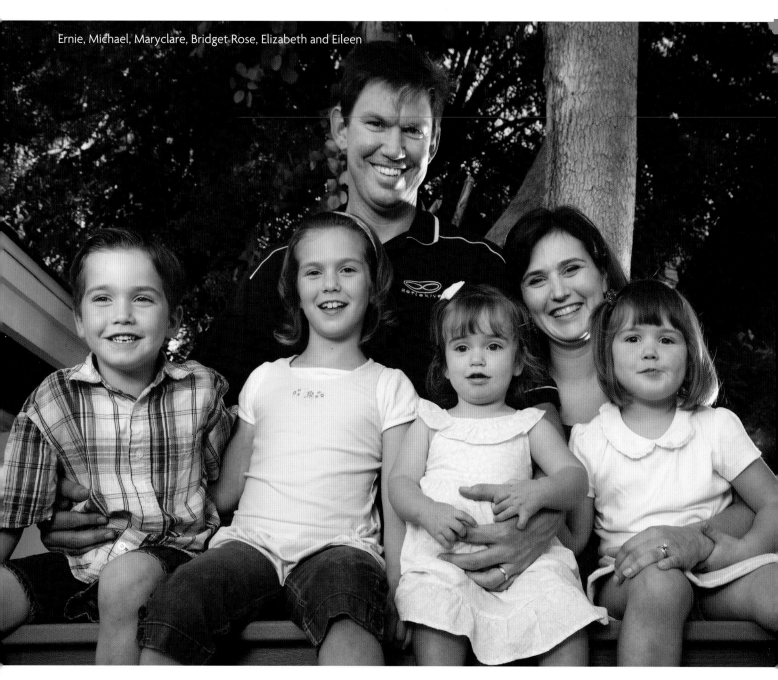

Ernie, Michael, Maryclare, Bridget Rose, Elizabeth and Eileen

One of the biggest challenges became parenting our other children, a one-year-old and a three-year-old. I had to leave them with others. Now I feel lucky that I get to be their full-time mom again.

Every time we asked for help, we got miles of help. So many people made sacrifices for us. Several took a leave of absence from work. Different organizations were fighting over who got to bring us meals. We needed them for so long that they all had a chance.

ERNIE, MARYCLARE'S FATHER: We've always been pretty strong Catholics, but this changed other people's faith. Some people said they didn't believe in prayer, but they were praying for Maryclare.

When we were just about to break, people started showing up at our door offering drastic measures to help. Sometimes it was just simple things. I came home one day and my grass was cut.

The community mobilization was the most impressive thing about all of this. You never know how many people you touch in your life until you hear from all of them in a ten-day period. And then you hear about all the people who aren't calling because everyone else is calling.

ELIZABETH: We developed an Internet care page where we could communicate with everyone. Masses were said in Italy, Germany, and Mexico for her. Friends of friends of friends. Because of the care page, they could keep up with intimate details. It wasn't just some story they heard.

> You never know how many people you touch in your life until you hear from all of them in a ten-day period.

Make-A-Wish Foundation built a beautiful tree house for Maryclare in our backyard. We thought it was going to be a couple of swings, and then they came and started pouring concrete. There are even lights and a doorbell.

She had the most amazing school and kindergarten teacher. Mrs. Adams would drive three hours every Saturday to the hospital and spend the whole day reading her stories and doing crafts. And she was a celebrity among her classmates.

What helped me the most was Maryclare's attitude. She found the bright side of everything. Even when she threw up, she was happy because she felt better. She kept cheering the rest of us on. After a month-long hospital stay, everything on the way home outside the car window was so exciting to her. It was such great medicine for her to get to come home for one night, touch her dolls, and put her head on her own pillow.

They told us after radiation and chemotherapy that she might be in a wheelchair. And then the miracle happened. In surgery, they opened her up and found nothing. No cancer. No one has offered any other explanation, other than a miracle. We had been praying harder than ever that the tumor would be dead. We were so impressed that God figured out an even better answer.

We've always been the kind of people who try to get as much as we can out of life, looking for opportunities for adventure, but we definitely do more so now. We don't sweat the small stuff. We realize a lot more that life is precious and we are so lucky to be the parents of these kids.

Matthew Zachary

Founder/CEO, Stupid Cancer, Inc.
Age at diagnosis, 21
Medulloblastoma, 1996

I was a senior in college and an intern at the World Trade Center when I began experiencing numbness in my hands. Not a good symptom for an aspiring concert pianist.

I returned to school and started playing piano, but I couldn't play as well. That was my first clue. The doctor said it was just carpal tunnel in my left arm. I slung my backpack on the other shoulder like he advised, but I still had problems.

I even had trouble gripping a pen. Doctors went down the line of possibilities—stroke, meningitis, Epstein-Barr, stomach virus—but they were clueless. By Thanksgiving break, my left hand was totally useless. I pleaded with doctors, "Can't I just finish the two weeks in the semester?" Ah, the ignorance of youth.

The symptoms kept getting worse, but I hid the blurred vision, fainting, slurred speech from my dad and most people. I finally went home, told my dad, and went in for an MRI. I was worried and confused about the mass they found in my cerebellum, but cancer didn't enter my mind.

In January 1996, I had a rare and risky surgery that removed the tumor. Four days later, I learned it was malignant. One bone marrow biopsy and three spinal taps showed I was clean. But since it was an unprecedented case and I was so young, there were no standards of treatment. The doctors couldn't reach a consensus.

I gained fifty pounds on steroids and then went through thirty-three days of high-intensity, full-body radiation. I then dropped 110 pounds in three months, lost the ability to swallow, and still had head pain. In spite of this, I managed to pass exams, graduate, compose music, write a musical, and play piano. I felt like a creative paraplegic.

Doctors were still recommending chemo. They said I'd be dead in five years with chemo and five and a half years without it. I did the math and opted not to do chemo. They have since determined that the chemo would have had no impact. I accidentally made the right choice.

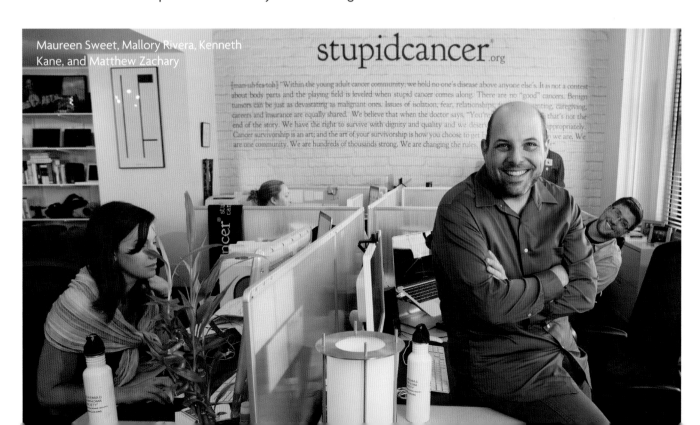

Maureen Sweet, Mallory Rivera, Kenneth Kane, and Matthew Zachary

At twenty-two, I had no life, no support and nowhere to go. No one gave advice about moving forward. That summer, I took a cross-country trip with my best friend and hiked the Grand Canyon. I had a bucket list before it was trendy.

When I returned home, I was depressed, unmotivated and scrawny. I had no therapy, no doctors, no follow-up. My father kept urging me to get a job, so I used the *New York Times,* scissors and a phone with a cord to find a job fixing computers. A year later, I moved out of my parents' house, became independent, and started writing music again.

In October of 1997, I decided to give a concert. About 100 people, including my coworkers, showed up, and I outed myself about my cancer. It was one big tear festival.

My real name is Matthew Zachary Greenswag, but Matthew Zachary became my new persona for my new life. In 2001, I threw a five-year anniversary "I'm not dead" party. That same year, I met a girl, started dating, and we're still married.

Over the next four years, I gave concerts at cancer events and began meeting other young people who had been through similar experiences.

In 2006, I learned that the five-year survival rates for young adults had remained flat since the 1970s, but the survival rate for older adults was skyrocketing because of increased cancer screening. This told me that there is an *age* issue to cancer. I realized that someone needed to be the voice of the millions of Millenniums who survived cancer.

I started "I'm Too Young For This" as a web resource. It wasn't about celebrity, ribbons, or contests. It was about giving survivors a sense of home and family and a voice with the right amount of disrespect and disruption. In 2007, our website was rated seventeen out of fifty in *Time Magazine*'s best websites list. After that, we started a radio show, formed chapters, and organized a conference. Everything from that point on became crowd-driven. We eventually changed the name to "StupidCancer.org."

We are still irreverent but respectful, and we've expanded to several conferences, a mobile app, boot camps, and meet-ups. We also serve young adults with parents who have cancer. The website and social media reach more than 33 million people a year.

Eighteen years later, I still have some chronic issues, but what can I do? Complain? I'm Jewish, so I do that anyway. I'm prone to blood cancer, have disintegrated capillaries, bipolar disorder, hyperthyroid, hormone issues, and permanent esophagitis. I'm on five meds; thankfully, none of them interact with each other.

> *"Everything that happens to you, whether you like it or not, becomes a part of your life. You must live your life and be the best you can be every step of the way."*

Through the miracle of sperm banking, my wife and I have beautiful twins who love to hear me play my music. When I was buried under a blanket, miserable and sick, I developed my mantra and wallpapered my bedroom with it: "Everything that happens to you, whether you like it or not, becomes a part of your life. You must live your life and be the best you can be every step of the way." That and the music got me through treatment and out of bed. That was my anchor.

Sorority Friends

Megan Berry
Age at diagnosis, 18
Thyroid cancer, 2006

Kelley Cohen
Age at diagnosis, 18
Biphenotypic leukemia, 2006

KELLEY: They found out I had a combination of two types of leukemia. Right off the bat, they wanted to do a bone marrow transplant. Out of four million people in the national bone marrow pool, I had eight matches and two perfect matches. I was so lucky. Someone I never knew saved my life. That's the most amazing gift in the world.

MEGAN: You don't ever think it's going to happen. My treatment was radiation, and then a year later, I had to do radiation again. I had so much radiation I had to be quarantined. And then this past summer, I had to have surgery to remove lymph nodes because they found cancer again.

The hardest part was watching my parents try to deal with it. I always knew I was going to make it through okay, no matter what. But watching them go through it was so awful. We are all very close. You could see the pain in their eyes.

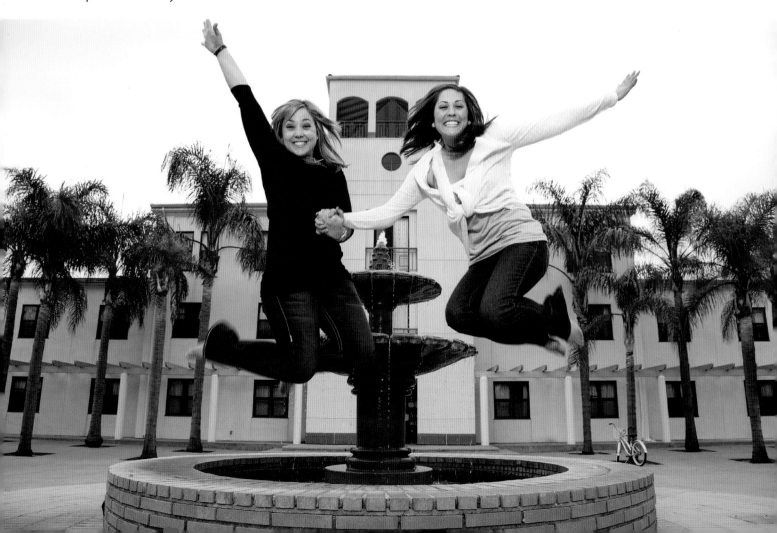

KELLEY: Two weeks after my diagnosis I sat down with my mom and cried. Then I said, "Okay, we've had our little pity party, now we will think positively." I aspire to be like my mother. Nothing gets her down. She is just incredible.

My dad and my brother and a bunch of his friends all shaved their heads for me. They actually beat me to it, so then I wanted my hair to fall out.

More than the cancer, I was upset to find out that I probably can't have babies. I always wanted to be a mom. I'm keeping hope, but if I can't, I'll adopt or explore other options.

MEGAN: Kelley and I became friends in the sorority even before we knew each other's stories. We immediately clicked and bonded because our families are so similar. I thought everyone had a family like mine, but we were tested and we found out just how special we really are.

KELLEY: I've learned to appreciate everything in my life, especially the people. I think I took my family for granted. My dad explained it best. He said that over all these years, we've been building a boat. You don't test the strength of the boat until you come up against a huge wave. We sure built a good boat.

MEGAN: It is the best-worst thing that ever happened to me. I learned at eighteen what most people take a lifetime to learn. My life was humming along, and the world was at my fingertips. And then it came to a screeching halt. I went numb.

> You don't test the strength of the boat until you come up against a huge wave.

When I was going into the operating room, they told me I had to stop crying or they couldn't do the surgery. And then I felt something touch me on the shoulder, but no one was there. It was a soft weight that made me very calm. Suddenly, I wasn't worried. In an instant something saved my life. Now I have a better perspective.

I wouldn't give it back if I could because I believe that everything happens for a reason, good or bad. When they told me the news, it was the worst day of my life. Everything after that got easier. It made me who I am, and I like the person I am today.

Kelley and I joke with each other . . . at eighteen we got it really bad, but at thirty-nine we'll be really healthy.

KELLEY: I graduated Loyola Marymount University as the valedictorian of my undergraduate class in 2011 and became an elementary teacher.

I have been cancer-free now for eight years. I have come to know my bone marrow donor and his family very well. His daughters are going to be junior bridesmaids in my upcoming wedding. Life is good.

MEGAN: One of my proudest moments is when I graduated from LMU in 2009, on time, with my original class. Walking across that stage was a thrill for me because of the added challenge of keeping up with the work during treatment. After graduation, the Muscular Dystrophy Association hired me as the Director of Business Development to raise money and awareness and plan events.

I love that what I do makes a difference. Because I was once on the other end of a scary diagnosis, being able to help those in their journey with MD is a powerful thing that I get to experience daily.

I've been cancer-free for eight years and going strong.

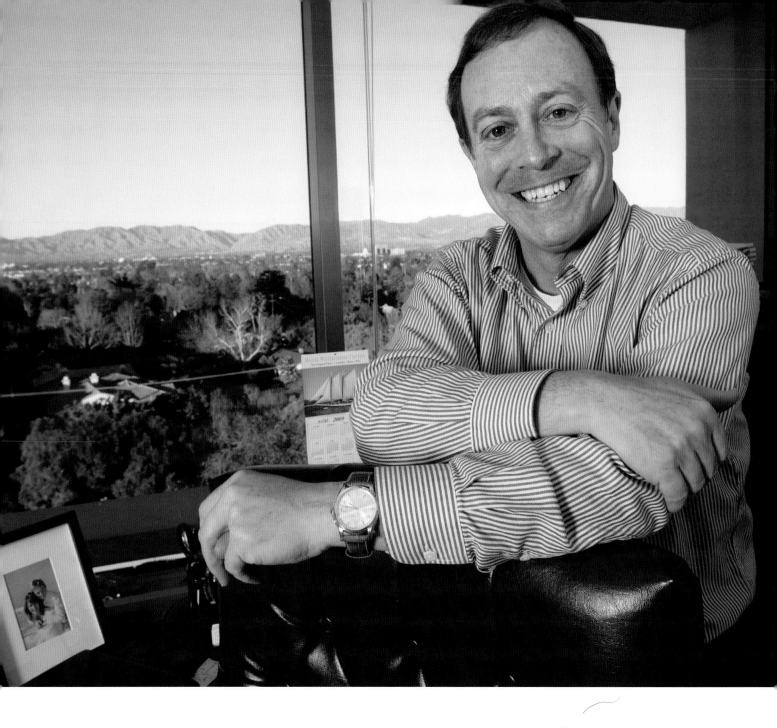

. . . I have learned that we might not choose our experiences, but we can choose how we adapt to them.

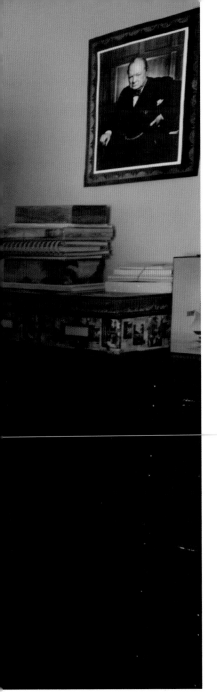

Michael Homier

| Attorney, Teacher (Business Law), Author
| Age at diagnosis, 20
| Testicular cancer, 1979

*W*hen I found out I had cancer at age twenty, I had to drop out of law school. It had a huge effect on my career, my self-image, and my relationship choices. I felt like damaged goods. I even married someone I shouldn't have because I thought no one else would have me. I hid my experience with cancer from everyone I met, even my close friends. I thought I was alone. I was mired in negativity for at least ten years.

I found out that this experience wasn't just mine. You're already in trouble as a teenager. You're already thinking weird things about yourself. And worse, you're already trying to let go of the people you love so you can fit in.

Teaching became an important part of my healing. I used to think that one person couldn't make a difference, and then I learned that's not true. I was making a difference. I couldn't deny it anymore. I was actually making a positive contribution. I had worth. The iceberg melted, and I finally began to take control. It lifted such a burden from my psyche.

Because of that, I have learned that we might not choose our experiences, but we can choose how we adapt to them.

My mission now is to offer myself as an example. I'd like to be someone I couldn't find back then, someone who can say to young people who are vulnerable, "You don't have to think that way. There's another way, and you *can* explore your dream."

When a doctor tells kids to go home because they're cured, they don't necessarily feel cured. I wish someone had told me when I left treatment about the emotional consequences of having cancer. I'd love to have those years back, but I can't. Perhaps though, I can help another person get through the transition.

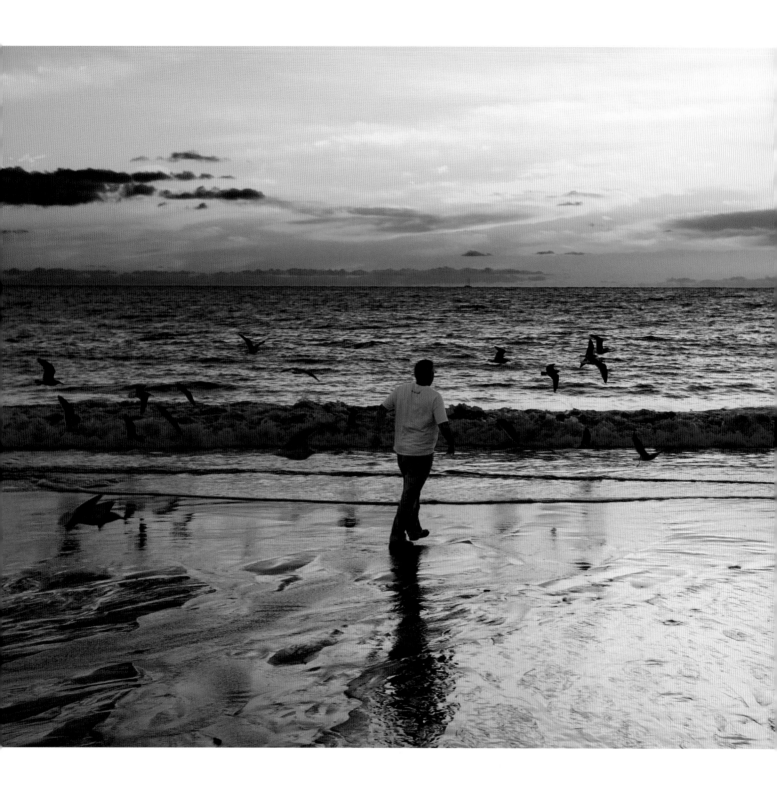

Once you're in the cancer club, and you get a chance to give a hand to someone else, make sure you do it.

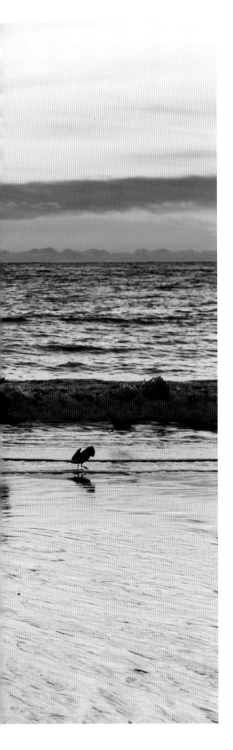

Michael Long

Satellite Launch Salesman
Age at first diagnosis, 39
Colon cancer, 2003
Cranial chondrosarcoma, 2006

*I*n 2003 I was flying internationally frequently on business, so I was constantly fatigued. I went to the doctor for a routine heart and lung checkup and, since everything looked good, I left for France the next day. When I walked into my hotel room, the phone was ringing. It was the doctor calling with my diagnosis. I flew home immediately, after first stopping on the way to the airport for a croissant, of course.

A colonoscopy revealed a tumor blocking a third of my colon. I immediately had surgery to remove the tumor, followed by six months of chemotherapy. The side effects were tough. I felt my life force draining from my body after each treatment. I slowly began the long road back to regain my strength. When I was getting chemo, I asked an oncology nurse why she did what she did. I did not expect her answer. She said that she is in this business because she gets to see the best of humanity.

Two years later in 2006, I was having double vision, and I went through several doctors before they discovered I had yet another tumor in my brain. It was a difficult case because the tumor was right in the middle of my head. Two days later, I got a call from a new doctor who said, "I think I can help you. Are you available to come in and talk?" And help he did. I had a very difficult and delicate surgery, followed by proton radiation. Once again, I came out okay.

Cancer helped me recalibrate myself. I was easygoing before, but these two experiences really changed my perspective on life. Now I always find the upside in every situation. Life is just . . . better. Only other cancer survivors would understand when I say that cancer is the best thing that can happen to you.

In December 2007, I had my third wake-up call: a car hit me. I made a T-shirt with nine cat faces and three of them are crossed out. The way I see it, I have my daughters who are the light of my life, and I still get to play soccer. That isn't too shabby.

My one message is that you *can* go through some terrible experiences and come out shining on the other end. Keep your head high, push through, and rely on the people that give you a hand. Once you're in the cancer club, and you get a chance to give a hand to someone else, make sure you do it. There is a joy that cannot be put into words in helping others. You cannot put a price tag on that feeling.

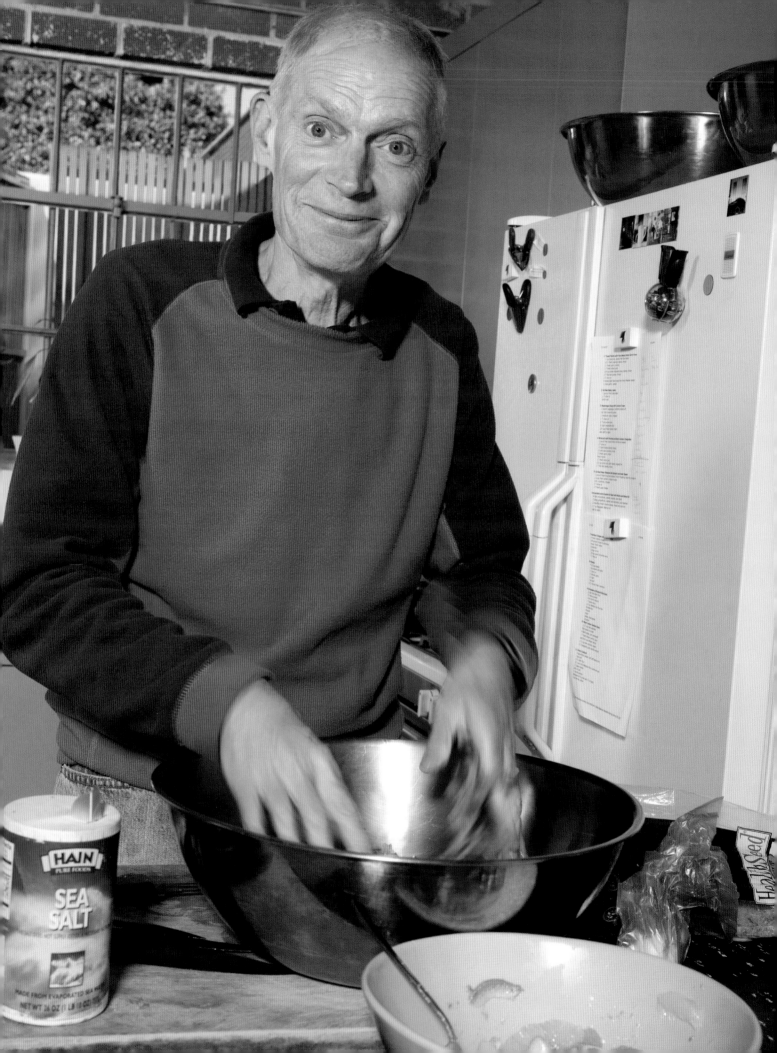

Michael Sieverts

Qi Gong Instructor
Age at diagnosis, 51
Malignant brain tumor, grade 3, 2000

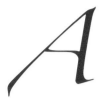t first they told me my seizures were panic attacks, and the doctors gave me antidepressants and tranquilizers. It's a measure of just how grim things were that I was happy when they discovered a brain tumor. My wife was weeping, and I thought it was great news.

I woke up paralyzed from surgery. It took me twenty-one days just to get out of the hospital.

Brain tumors are their own weird and confusing thing. Your brain is your self, your soul, and your identity. And when it gets damaged, you still have to use your brain to make decisions about your brain. It gets very confusing.

The role of the caregiver becomes critical. There's no other way to describe it except that I became stupid after my surgery. We had to have Post-its around the house saying things like "Stove on?" And, trust me: It's not easy being stupid. The little one-year-old boy next door and I learned to walk and tie our shoes together.

Now after various treatments, I am fully functional. It is so good to have my cognition back.

I give enormous credit to my doctors: my neurosurgeon and radiation oncologist, and my long-term neuro-oncologist. Having doctors as skilled as they were was very important. I also believe, however, that the acupuncture, physical therapy, nutrition changes, meditation practice, support groups, along with Qi Gong, were hugely beneficial.

I had been in commercial real estate, a tense and cutthroat world—not the right place for me to be while I dealt with regaining my strength and cognition. I had to learn to deal with my cancer on a subtle, internal level, almost like having a direct conversation with it. Intellectually, I feel that I must also have that subtle relationship with everything I put in my body. For example, cooking for me is not just about the food. It's also about taking control, taking care of who I am and using my dollars to vote for a healthy and sustainable food system.

I feel like my life started when I had my seizure. I used to hear people say that their life-threatening illness was the best thing that ever happened to them. I thought they were crazy. But the reality is, this really is the best thing that ever happened to me. The most terrifying thing in the world happened, and I'm okay.

The most terrifying thing in the world happened, and I'm okay.

Michelle Swaney

Full-Time Mom
Age at diagnosis, 24
Colon cancer, stage 2, 2006

MICHELLE: When they told me I had cancer, I started laughing in my head and thought, *Uh-hah! See, it wasn't just cramps.* I was relieved that there was a reason for all the pain. Then they handed me a pamphlet from the American Cancer Society, and I said, "Well this is ironic. I helped edit that." This time, I looked for more than poor grammar.

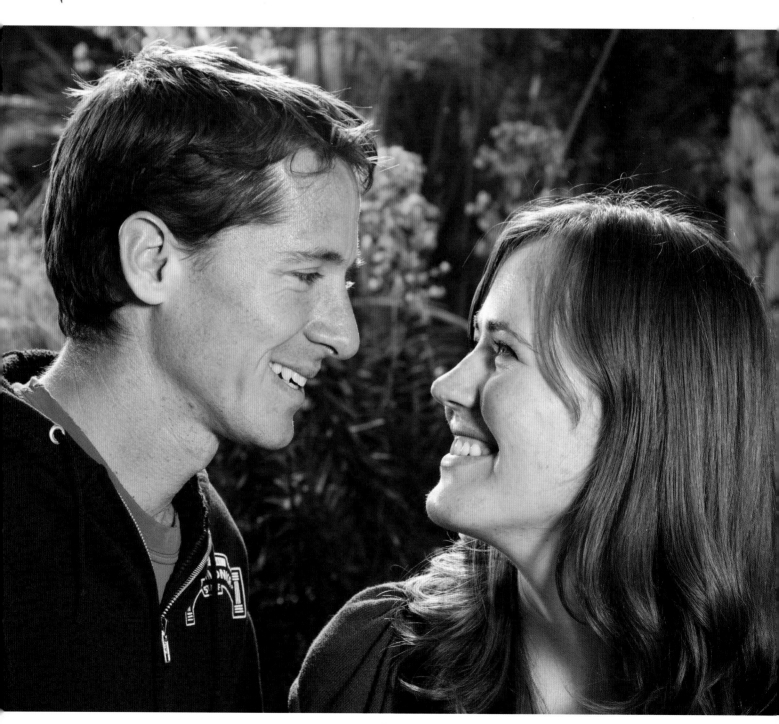

The doctors immediately started talking about surgery, chemo-therapy, and freezing my eggs. The discussion brought up all kinds of moral decisions that were difficult to deal with. I prayed a lot, and I cried a lot. A question that I had to confront concerning chemotherapy was, "Would I rather be a healthy mom to adopted children or an unhealthy mom to my own biological children?" I decided that I would rather be healthy for any children that God blessed me with.

I decided that I would rather be healthy for any children that God blessed me with.

The day after my surgery, my future boyfriend, Matt, literally brought me the ocean. Even though my hospital room looked out on the beach, I couldn't see it from my bed, so he filled a bowl with sand, seashells, and water.

MATT: Cancer is an intense thing to deal with when starting a relationship. I worried about what kind of signals I was sending. Then I decided I wasn't going to avoid something good for someone just because of what she might think. Eventually, I learned that God wanted me to be there for Michelle. But it was hard for me to recognize that I couldn't do everything. I couldn't heal her.

MICHELLE: It took a while for the relationship to develop, partly because barfing is not really romantic. And then one day he watched when they were sticking a tube up my nose, and he looked at me like I was still a pretty person. He was there with me through everything. I remember thinking *if we were to get married, I wouldn't have to worry about his vow 'in sickness and in health.'*

I was also lucky that I had a supportive boss and many others who wanted to help. Seeing other people's strengths was the best thing for me. I learned that I had limitations and I needed to ask for help. If you don't, you won't see the best in people. I had to let go and tell people things like, "It would really be nice if you could get me soup."

I also tried to figure out how my cancer could be a positive influence on others. You can be in a bad situation and be sad, or you can search for the good. I tried to spread that good to everyone. It's intense for someone my age to be around people who are dying, but it became the most important thing in my life. Suddenly, nothing else mattered more than what I was learning from them. It occurred to me that I wouldn't have even met them if I hadn't had cancer.

I have always thought it would be harder to watch someone go through cancer than to actually go through it myself. After I was diagnosed, I learned that was true. I could see the pain in the eyes of my family. It brought up a lot of emotions, but that made us all closer. Who would think that cancer could be such a healer?

Matt and I have been happily married since 2009. We now have one child, a fifteen-month-old boy, and I am pregnant with our second, due in March 2014. We have been blessed with these children naturally, without having to undergo medical interventions. Matt and I also recently became certified through "Safe Families for Children" to temporarily host children whose parents are going through difficult times, including cancer treatment. According to my oncologist (as of 2012) I am considered "medically cured." He said he now only wants to see me in our yearly family Christmas cards.

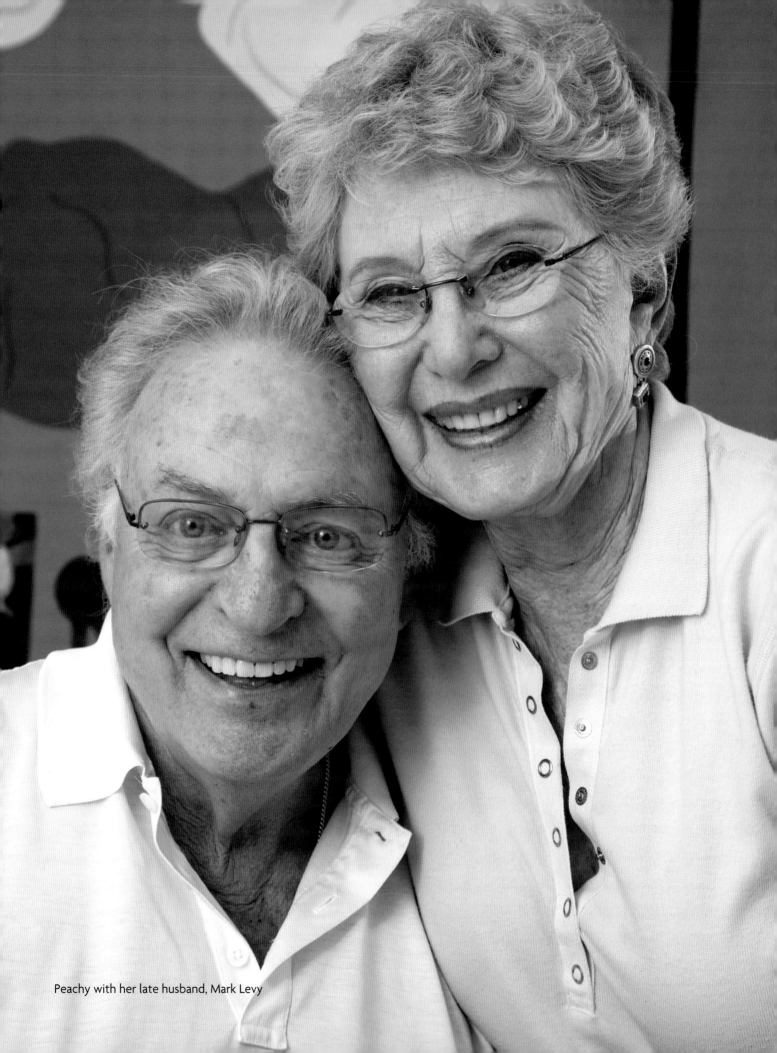

Peachy with her late husband, Mark Levy

Peachy Levy

Artist, Wife, Mother, Grandmother
Age at diagnosis, 74
Breast cancer, 2004

I never thought a thing like cancer would happen to me. My body works too well. I've heard other people's stories, but in my heart of hearts, it wasn't going to happen to me. I wouldn't get breast cancer. I'm not a worrier, and if I have any worries, they are more about my husband than myself.

When I heard that indeed I had breast cancer, I was more surprised than fearful. On the day I was diagnosed, the doctor told me that it was very early and that he could remove it all without having to remove any lymph nodes. Because the surgery was going to be early the next morning, I didn't have time to worry.

I haven't always understood my inner strength. When I was younger I didn't have much self-confidence. My husband helped me to understand my value. He encouraged me to undertake many activities and to do them well. And then

I have been married to the love of my life for 64 years. We adore each other.

years later, I said to myself, *I only have so much time here. And so while I still have my hands and my eyes, and my spiritual resonance, I want to accomplish more in the artistic field that I have chosen.* So I have done a lot of reevaluating of my life since my diagnosis and made choices that allowed me more time to do what has brought me great satisfaction.

Cancer has not changed my feeling that I will live a long life.

I have been very fortunate. I have a wonderful family and I have been married to the love of my life for 64 years. We adore each other.

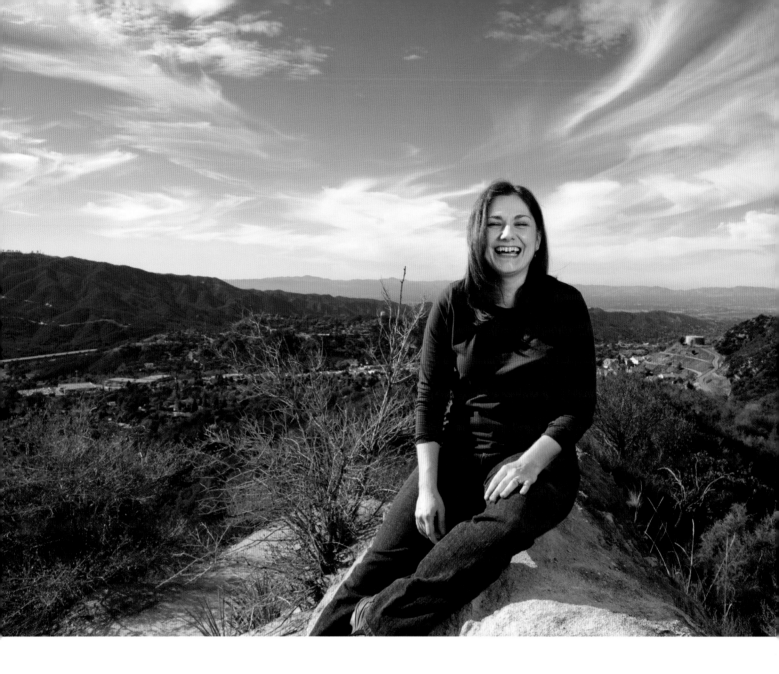

It's about joy, about living our soul's purpose, and about contributing to the greater good. I live every moment with that in mind.

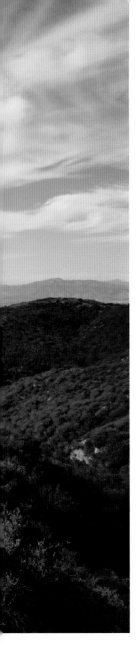

Rebecca Gifford

Writer
Age at diagnosis, 22
Non-Hodgkin's lymphoma, 1994
Recurrence, 1995

I was living in Cincinnati right after college when I was diagnosed with lymphoma. All I heard in my head was, *You're twenty-two and you have cancer.* How do you process that? I did chemotherapy and radiation, but a year later it re-infested in my kidney, so I had to endure another round of chemo and a bone marrow transplant.

After that, I didn't have a focus anymore. There was no way to reason it all out. At the time, that bothered me a lot. Everyone around me was so happy that I got through the treatments and could get back to normal. They didn't realize that there was no more normal.

I was young and still trying to figure out who I was and who I wanted to be. Then cancer changed everything. From then on, I was looking through a different-colored window because my perspective and direction dramatically shifted.

The greatest initial impact was that I became much less fearful of risk. I had conquered something big, so I was willing to do things that were not necessarily comfortable for me or for the people around me. I just stood up and said, "I want to become a writer," moved to New York City, and joined a group of struggling artists. I never imagined doing that before cancer.

Romantically, however, I felt like damaged goods. Cancer is the ultimate conversation stopper. At that age, hardly anyone you date has dealt with mortality. When do you tell them that you had cancer and can't have children? Most people in their twenties slowly become more comfortable with their identities, but something like this will quickly make you come of age. I had faced death, and I gained a big-picture perspective. I was fortunate to have learned all of that so early in life.

My diagnosis presented me with the clarity I needed to see the path I was supposed to be on, and my survival gave me the courage to follow that path. I was given the opportunity to live this life more fully, in a way that is probably very different than it would have been. I'm happy, and I greet both the challenges and the opportunities life brings. My husband and I adopted a beautiful child, and our little family has moved all over the country with the inherent freedom and strength to go where life takes us.

My life doesn't meet everyone's expectations, but that matters so much less than it used to. My parents used to want me to have a job they could explain and a title they could understand. But when my book came out (*Cancer Happens: Coming of Age with Cancer*), they understood what I do and why. Life is about so much more than traditional success. It's about joy, about living our soul's purpose, and about contributing to the greater good. I live every moment with that in mind.

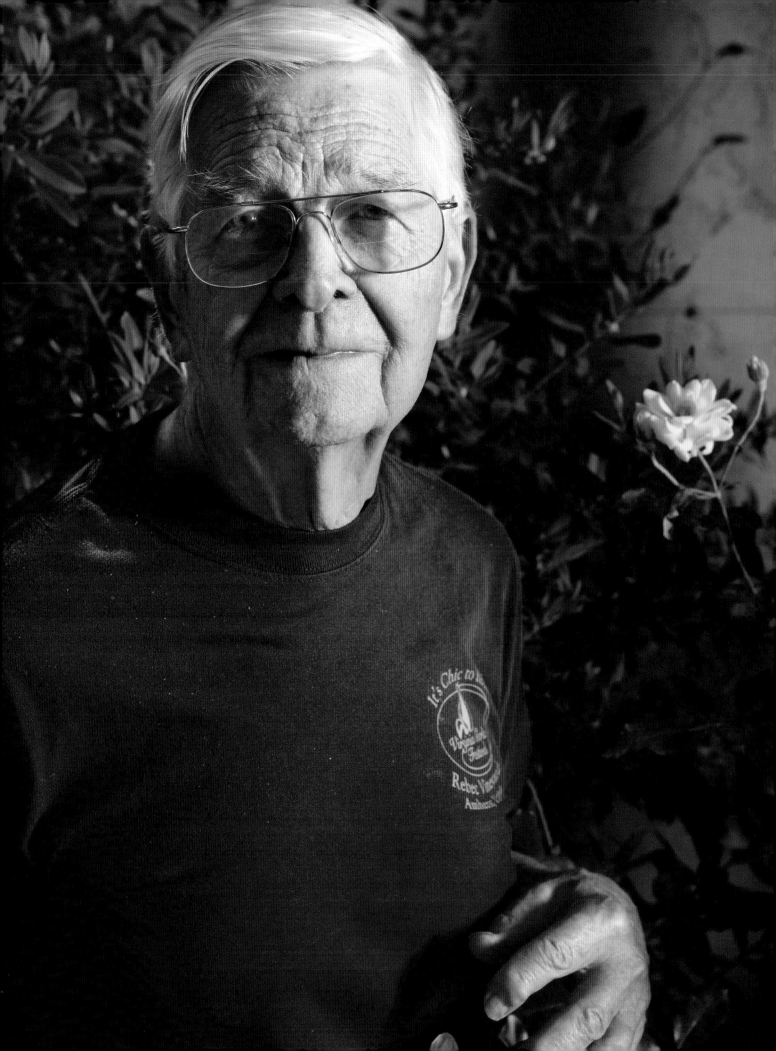

Richard Hanson

Chemical Engineer, Farmer, Winemaker, Rebec Vineyards
Age at diagnosis, 64
Bladder cancer, 1988
Recurrence, 2005

I believe that our lives continues after we die, biologically through our children and then in so many other ways through what we have done for others. If there is any way I can be of help to someone else, I am always willing to do that. When you help others, there is no question it helps you more.

Cancer makes us more aware of our mortality and the fragility of our life. Having cancer is not what I call a blessing, but I can tell you, since cancer I've had a ball. A week after my operation I was dancing at my vineyard's garlic festival.

I'm so happy to be alive. I'm aware of what life means and what a great thing life is, but also how tenuous and fragile it is. We should all live every day as if it is our last. So I dance . . . not necessarily more than I used to, but I sure don't dance less. I'm trying to build a new facility on my own property for dancing so I don't have to go very far.

These are the best years of my life.

When you help others, there is no question it helps you more.

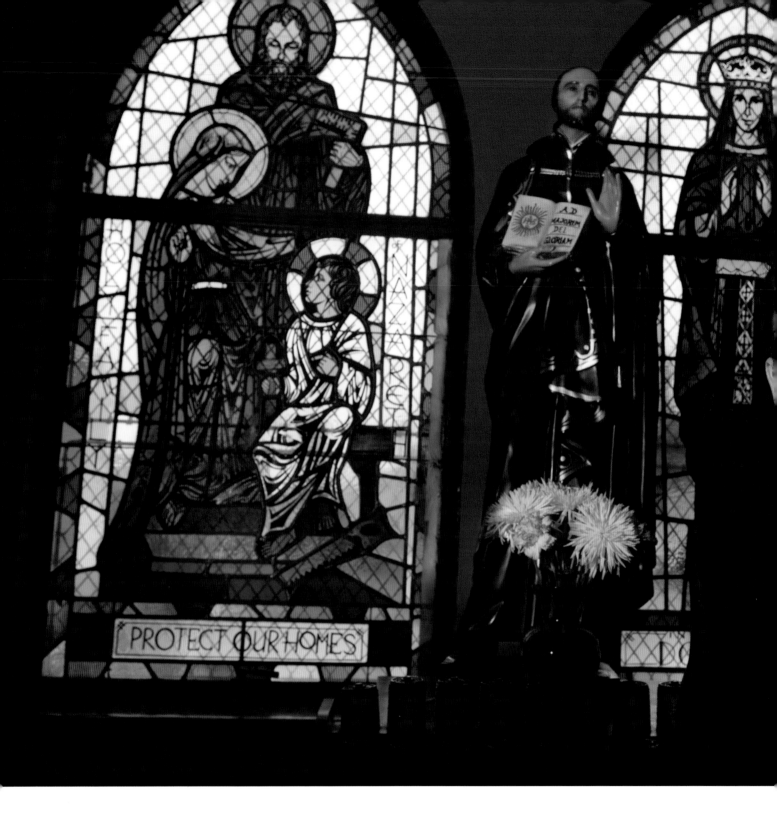

The people that survive are the ones who know they have to fight.

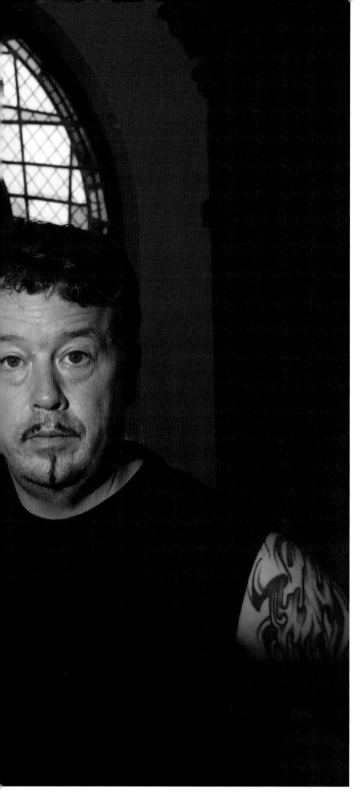

Robert Crozier

Retail Management
Age at diagnosis, 49
Liver cancer, 1999
Recurrence, 2008

*I*t seems like I've spent a lifetime jumping over hurdles. I grew up really poor and had a heart infection as a teenager. As an adult, I was homeless for a while and for many years abused my body with drugs. I have also experienced a lot of family difficulties.

Cancer is just another one of the stumbling blocks in my life that I had to jump over. You can't stand up and say, "Poor me." There is a switch that turns on inside of you to be positive; you have to turn off the switch for pity or weakness. The people that survive are the ones who know they have to fight.

During chemo, a light bulb went off in my head. I realized that I had to endure getting to the brink of death after each treatment and yet keep my spirits up, my energy up, and my health up. I had to realize that there would be a light at the end of the tunnel.

Cancer gave me a sense of mortality. I am not nearly as concerned about material things. I also don't think about aging anymore. Who knows if I'll make it? I think about today, and I don't take anything for granted.

If you give back to the system what you take, assume that most people are good, and treat everyone as a friend, you learn that there is plenty out there for everyone.

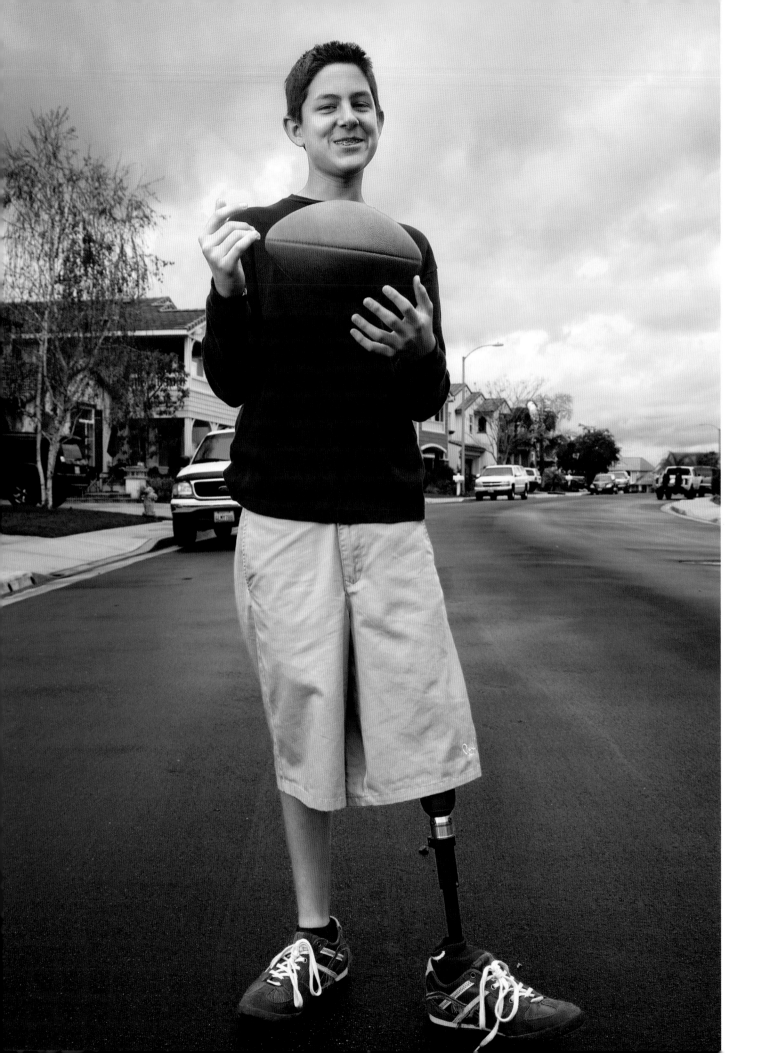

Robert Ram | Age at diagnosis, 12
Ewing's sarcoma, 2006

RAVI, ROBERT'S FATHER: After six rounds of chemo, Robert had a knee replacement. His lower leg did not take it well and started to die. Over the course of two weeks, he was in and out of the operating room nine times. The final option was amputation. He then had to have three more rounds of chemo.

LIIA, ROBERT'S MOTHER: You hear stories and never think about it happening to your own family. It was a struggle, but we knew we had to be strong. It was hard for our other kids. It affected their schoolwork. Our whole life was upside down because we were spending so much time at the hospital. But all this adversity and chaos brought us so much closer.

ROBERT: When the doctor told me I had cancer, I knew immediately that my life was going to change, but I didn't know how. Since then, I've gotten to do amazing things and meet amazing people. I got to be on the field and announce the line-up for the Anaheim Angels at one of their games. And I went to a running clinic with Paralympic athletes who taught me how to run.

RAVI: He has always been an athlete, so now he just has to find a new outlet. We don't know what that is just yet, but in addition to the running, he's already an umpire for Little League. Many others who have lost limbs have told him that they wish they had had his spirit.

I know that he's destined to do something amazing and change people. He shows off his prosthetic leg like it's a prize. When little kids stare at his leg, he has them come over and touch it and ask questions. Then he teases them and scratches it like it's itching. He has such a good sense of humor about it. Some days he'll put a Band-Aid on it.

ROBERT: Parents tell their kids not to touch it, and I always say, "Go ahead. It's okay." People feel like they can't be honest with me now because it's going to hurt my feelings. I wish everyone would just tell me the truth. I don't like being treated differently.

LIIA: Robert graduated from high school in 2013, having earned a varsity letter for swimming and water polo. He is attending a local junior college, with the hopes of transferring to the University

We don't look back. Only forward.

of California at Irvine in two to three years for a bachelor's degree in computer programming. He is an active mentor and speaker for the Challenged Athletes Foundation and has spoken at many local schools about adversity and never giving up. He is also training to swim for the 2016 Paralympics in Brazil. He has two national cut times and is hoping to make the US team by the summer of 2014 so that he can begin competing at an international level.

He proves to all of us that you can always make the best of anything. We quickly realized how precious life is. We could have lost one of our children. So now we tell them all to live every day because you never know what tomorrow might bring. We don't look back. Only forward.

Robert Stepp

Age at diagnosis, 3
Ewing's sarcoma, 2007

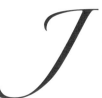ANIE, ROBERT'S MOTHER: Robert had a great summer playing soccer and swimming, and then a few days after a fun day at a carnival, he went into respiratory arrest. Five days later, the doctors discovered a tumor so severe they couldn't figure out a way to even do a biopsy. In a very scary moment, we decided to have them do surgery. They found cancer.

DOYLE, ROBERT'S FATHER: We entered an entirely new world. When you arrive on the pediatric cancer floor of the hospital, the kids just want to run and have fun. But as parents, you might as well be landing on a beach in Normandy.

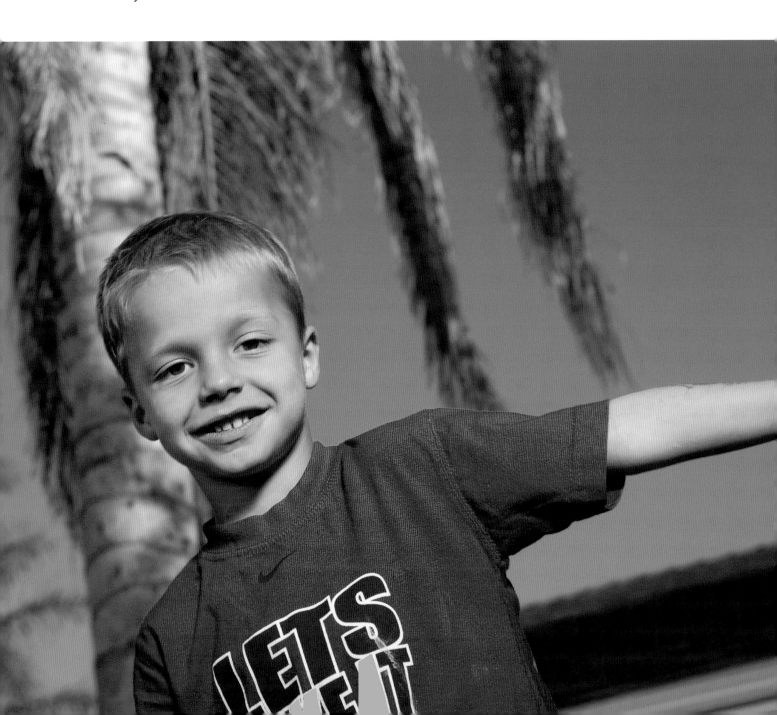

We then went through fourteen cycles of severe chemotherapy for nine months, another surgery in the middle of it, and then seven weeks of radiation every day. At the end of all of the treatments, the lowest point was when the doctors told me that Robert still had cancer and it would take a miracle to save his life.

JANIE: All of a sudden, he was in total remission. That was when I really broke down and cried. Robert asked me, "Mommy, why are you crying?" I hugged him and said, "Happy tears, honey, happy tears." The boy has never calmed down since then. He is constantly on the go. It's a true blessing to have him bouncing around now.

ROBERT: Look at my scars. Now I'm a man! They made my tumor glow and then they threw it in the dirty trash.

DOYLE: We were always trying to think of ways to make it fun and keep him from being scared. One day the doctors told me that he would probably have red urine that night. I pointed to his red IV bag and said, "Guess what? That stuff they are putting into you right now is going to make you pee like Superman!" He went to bed so excited, woke up to pee around 11:00 p.m., and then started crying. "It's not red. I'm not Superman."

When his blood counts were low, he would show his pain by getting aggressive. One evening in the hospital, I heard he was hitting his mother that day. I took him, dragging his IV pole behind him, to the stairwell, because that was the only place we could have privacy. I told him that if he wanted to hit someone, he should hit me. He swung his arm back as far as he could and slapped my face. I then asked him, "When you hit Mommy and Daddy, do you think it makes us feel good?" He looked at me for a second, burst out crying, and gave me a big hug.

Look at my scars. Now I'm a man!

JANIE: We were not a religious family, and so it shocked me one day in the hospital when Robert started talking to God. He told me that He was in the room. I was afraid to leave him for fear that God was going to take him. I was petrified to ask Robert details. Eventually I took comfort in knowing that God was in the room or, as a friend told me, that He was there so that I could step away.

Robert asked me to take him to the hospital chapel so he could pray. He knelt down and said, "God, please take this cancer out of me and make my mommy happy again." From then on, no one will ever be able to tell me that God does not exist. Believe it or not, Doyle and I eventually became Sunday school teachers.

DOYLE: Throughout history, fathers abandoned their families during a tragedy. It wasn't because they didn't love them; it was because they lost their roles. They felt helpless. This tragedy drove us apart, and then it brought us back again so much closer. We saw qualities in each other that we hadn't seen before. I wanted our family to survive.

JANIE: From now on, my family will always come first. Before all of this, I wanted to be a vice president at work. Now I don't give a damn. I'm not in the rat race any longer. I had to sit down and tell my bosses that they were not number one anymore. I love my job, but I will not put my family on the back burner.

DOYLE: The photograph in my office and the vision I will always remember is Robert with a bald head, a sunken face, an IV coming out of his chest, and he's in the hospital playroom break dancing.

ROBERT: I married five nurses while I was there!

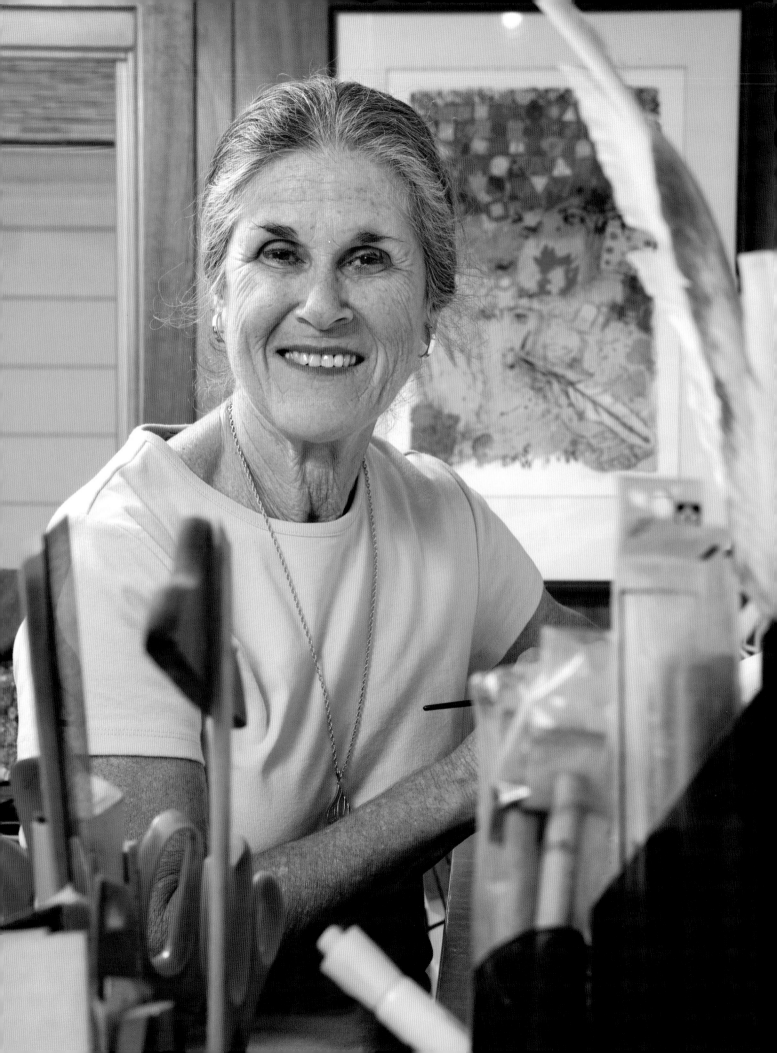

Ruth Merritt

Artist
Age at first diagnosis, 62
Pancreatic cancer, 1997
Lung cancer, 2001; recurrence, 2003

When I was diagnosed with pancreatic cancer sixteen years ago, my first reaction was "Why me?" That lasted about ten seconds. I wanted to get to the next step and do what I had to do. My children went to the Internet and asked if I wanted to know what they found. I said "no." The only thing I wanted to know was what I needed to do to get from today to tomorrow. I didn't want more truth than I could handle. When you have to be upbeat, the last thing you need is all the stuff you don't need to know.

That worked for me. I'm glad I didn't find out that the prognosis for pancreatic cancer was so dire. Instead, I went on with my life. Three and a half years later, I had to have surgery again for lung cancer. Shortly after that I was climbing to the top of the Duomo in Italy, minus one lobe. I also went back to playing tennis, and I'm still playing.

The artwork I do is based on Hebrew letters and symbolism. And yet I question if there is really a God. If there is a God, I don't think He's one that sits there and answers individual prayers. On the tennis courts some people pray before they hit a ball. If God is busy with everybody's tennis, no wonder the world is screwed up. I don't think I would pray to that God.

Instead, I do my artwork because it's upbeat and happy work. I'm not a person who holds everything inside and pours it out in my art. I'm a talker. When I'm finished talking, there's nothing left to pour out.

I think I've always been in touch with my feelings, so that didn't have to change after cancer. I always tell it like it is, and I don't beat around the bush or mince words. But telling it like it is has its problems. Not everyone wants a straight answer, so I've learned to be a little gentler. I haven't become totally diplomatic; I would never get a post in an embassy anywhere. Now I ask, "Do you really want me to talk about it, or do you want me to listen?"

I learned a lot from my support system, and that understanding changed how I behave with other people. I have more sensitivity to others. I kept track of every donation and honor card and a list of every phone call. At heart, I'm really sentimental. I'm a crybaby. I really am. Just don't tell anybody.

Now I ask, "Do you really want me to talk about it, or do you want me to listen?"

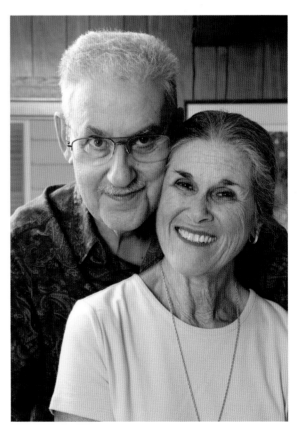

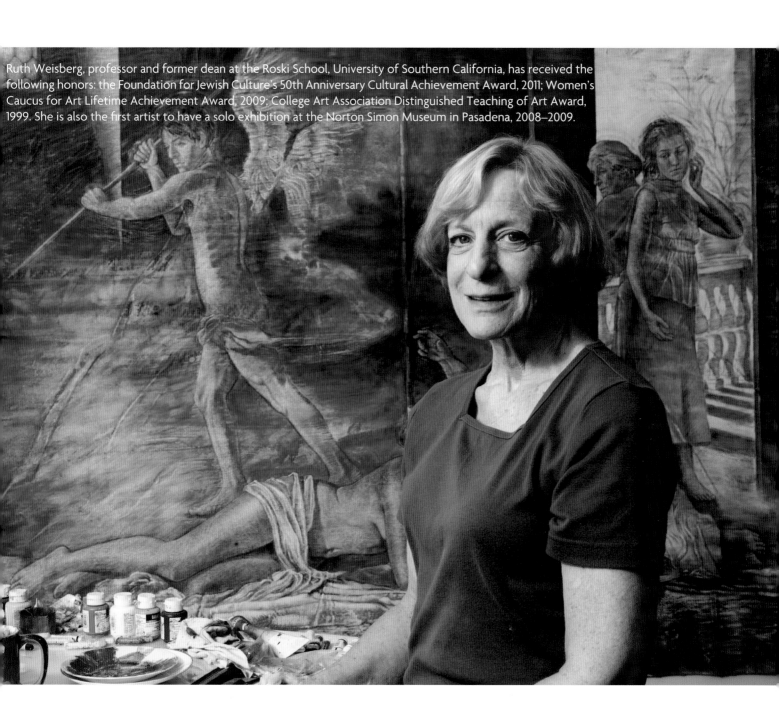

Ruth Weisberg, professor and former dean at the Roski School, University of Southern California, has received the following honors: the Foundation for Jewish Culture's 50th Anniversary Cultural Achievement Award, 2011; Women's Caucus for Art Lifetime Achievement Award, 2009; College Art Association Distinguished Teaching of Art Award, 1999. She is also the first artist to have a solo exhibition at the Norton Simon Museum in Pasadena, 2008–2009.

Ruth Weisberg

Artist, Professor of Art, Roski School of Fine Arts, University of Southern California
Age at first diagnosis, 41
Breast cancer, 1983; recurrence, 1986

I was shocked when I got my breast cancer diagnosis after my first mammogram. I was in my early forties and felt great. I went through a round of treatment and was told I only had a ten percent chance of a recurrence. But someone has to be in that ten percent. When the cancer recurred, I was frightened for a few years, but I've gone on to a very active life. I want other patients to see that cancer is not a death sentence and that lingering effects are often minor.

When I was going through treatment, I found that some people were absolutely wonderful in their support. That strengthened our friendship. Others were frightened and didn't want to see me. I now try to make as many phone calls as I can, even to people I don't know personally, to tell them that there can be a great life after their diagnosis and treatment.

With breast cancer, there is a sense of loss due to a change in your womanhood. Each woman's experience is different, but there is always an internal trauma concerning perceived image. A portion of that is very real, but a huge part is psychological. The loss is more anxiety than reality. Physical benefits can actually occur. It takes a little courage to relearn your body sexually and discover new avenues of pleasure. It can be even better than before.

Cancer has an added benefit of making life itself more precious. Someone might not choose to have that benefit, but it is accompanied by a shift in your mindset toward your blessings. Our most profound gifts are completely inexpressible. I've seen some people shut down, while many others choose to live life more fully.

My art sustained me through everything. There is a trajectory and an emotional tenor in my work reflecting loss, but there is also a heightened sense of life as a result of those losses. In many of my paintings, someone is leaving, which gives my art a feeling of moving forward. I have a lineage as an artist based on capturing an essential humanness and being in dialogue with history. For me, it is clear who I am—I know my voice. It may sound complicated, but most things that are interesting are complex.

> *My art sustained me through everything.*

I feel like I was prepared for loss because Judaism prepares us for that; this one, however, was closer and was more about my own mortality. When you are in your early forties, you envision yourself as someday being an eighty or ninety-year-old. And then suddenly something happens, and that vision vanishes for a while.

In a monumental ninety-four-foot-long piece, *The Scroll*, done in the mid-eighties, I began to develop an image of a river of souls. The possibility of death implied a kind of continuity with everyone who had gone before me. I feel that there is a total circle of life, which is a summary of all of my work as an artist. Even thirty years later, that image of a river of souls reappears in my work from time to time. It is always there below the surface.

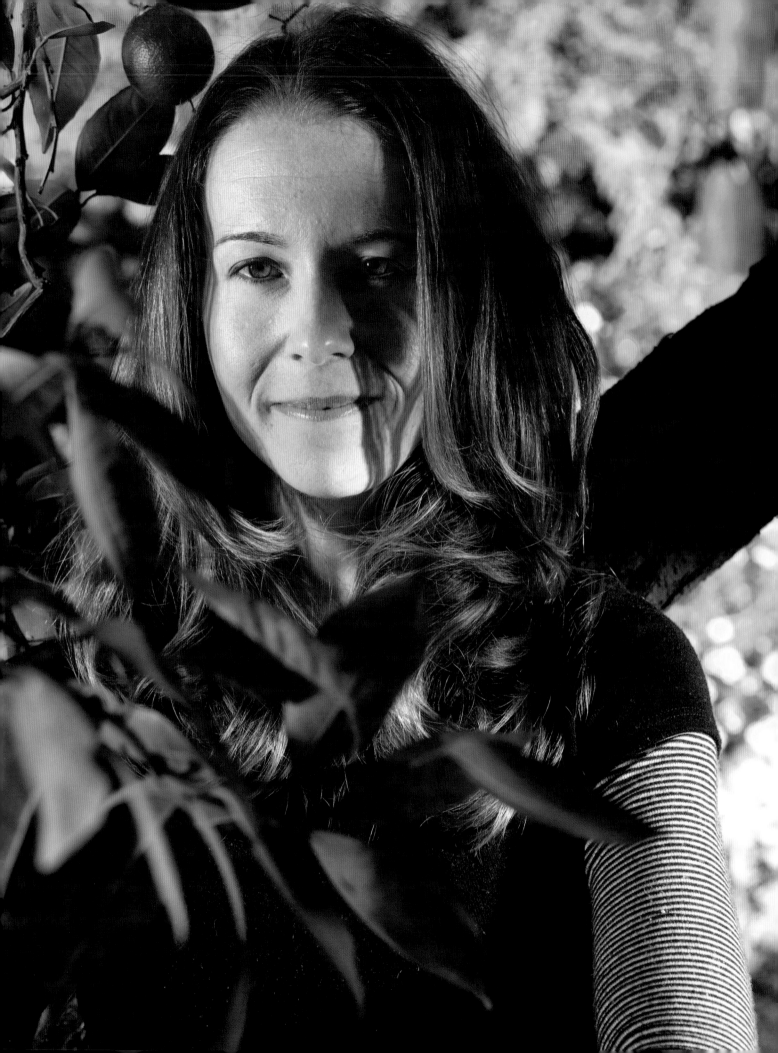

Sabrina Dossi Mansfield

Producer, Director for Film and Video
Age at diagnosis, 28
Squamous cell carcinoma of the tongue, 2005
Recurrence, 2006

SABRINA: By the time I was diagnosed, the cancer had spread from my tongue to several levels of lymph nodes in my neck. I was just out of graduate school, healthy and active, and my career was just starting to take off—I couldn't figure out how this could possibly be happening. I didn't know anyone my age who had been through anything like this. My oncologist explained that at my age, this particular cancer would be aggressive . . . he was right.

Life changed instantly; I was now a full-time cancer patient. I had to make the appointments, get second opinions, third opinions, holistic advice, biopsies, scans and more scans, and deal with my insurance. Sometimes, I had to be very firm and demand my treatments. One procedure took eighteen phone calls. Meanwhile, I was producing an elaborate music video that I refused to abandon ship on.

When I first learned I had cancer, my husband Max and I had only been dating for eight months. Before I told him, I prepared myself: "This might be it for us, he might choose not to stick around and you *have* to be ready to accept that." Not only did he stick by my side through everything, but he was relentlessly making me laugh with his wild and irreverent humor. He was amazing. I learned how much stamina and strength he has. I think about our relationship all the time and how fortunate I am to have him in my life.

MAX, SABRINA'S HUSBAND: From the very beginning, Dossi recognized that this would also be very difficult for me. She decided that no matter how bad she felt or how hard things got, she wasn't going to use me as her solitary crutch or as her punching bag. I really appreciated that. She recognized that it wasn't fair for me, because there was nothing I could do. From my standpoint, it was like being in a war and watching from the back lines while she was up at the front.

SABRINA: My cancer came back less than a year later. The first round I was so angry because the cancer had stopped my life and kept me from pursuing my dreams. I spent the first round making an enemy of the situation. For the second round, I decided I was not going to live that life again. I had to stop fighting it and accept that, for the moment, this was my life. From there, I could decide that getting treatments was a *good* thing and that I was going to survive. Even on my way to getting multiple tubes surgically implanted into my neck for internal radiation, I was skipping down the hallway.

> For the second round, I decided I was not going to live that life again.

The personal shifts in my life have been due to self-exploration—not necessarily due to cancer, but perhaps heightened by it. I still have a strong sense of being grateful, just as I did before. I've never really sweated the small stuff. Other people have told me I've been an inspiration, and I try to be an ally to others who are going through what I went through. Above all, living in the now instead of fighting it, is the most important goal in my life. Max and I now have two beautiful boys together, one biological and one foster/adopted. Max continues to make me laugh every day.

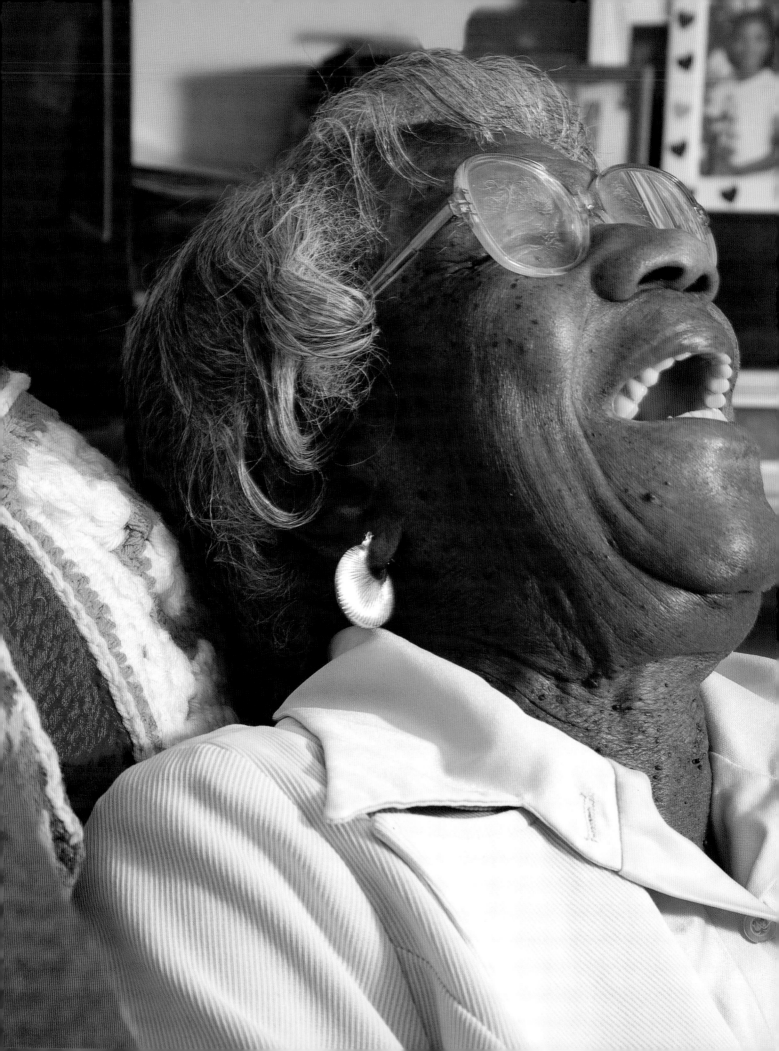

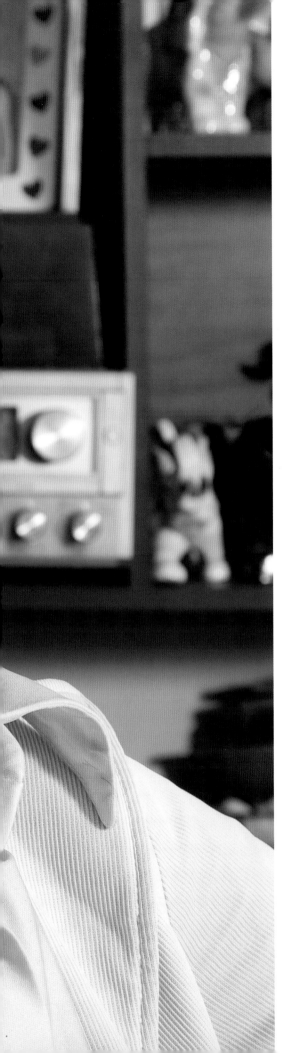

Sally Craigen

Centenarian
Age at first diagnosis, 64
Breast cancer, 1972
Ovarian cancer, 2001

I am a two-time cancer survivor, but I never stopped enjoying life—dancing and singing with the choir. I'm still singing today.

People would always say to me, "Sally, you don't act like you have cancer." Yes, I'm hurting sometimes, but not enough to stop *enjoying* life.

Yes, I'm hurting sometimes, but not enough to stop enjoying life.

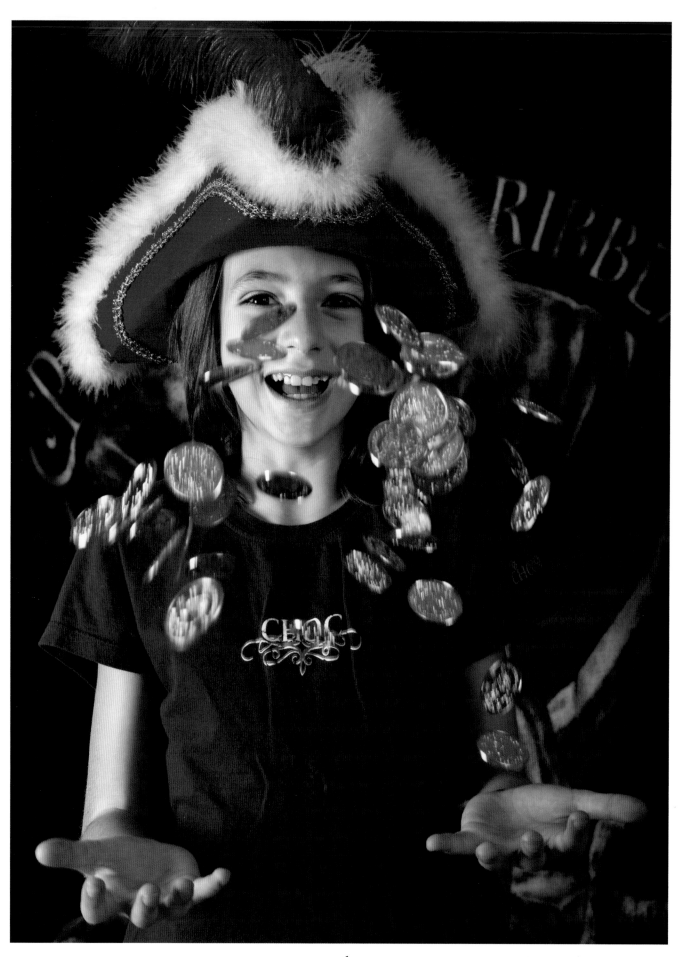

Samantha Heim

Age at diagnosis, 8
Late stage Rabdomyosarcoma in
salivary gland area, 2006; diagnosed
in only 300 children per year

E RIN, SAMANTHA'S MOM: Before Sammy was diagnosed, my husband and I lived in a Pollyannaish world. When Sammy got sick, we didn't consider cancer a possibility at all. When she was admitted to the hospital and we took her to the room, we saw that we were on the oncology floor. Rich looked at me and said, "I guess they didn't have room on the other floors." I never imagined we'd fall into this world of cancer. We soon learned differently.

Cancer doesn't just happen to you. It happens to the whole family. The very first thing I did after she was diagnosed was to send an email to my entire address book: "All I'm asking is that you send this to all of your friends to get a prayer chain going that will wrap around the world."
Without our faith, we could not have gotten through this.

SAMANTHA: I knew it was a really bad sickness, and kids could die. But I didn't, and eventually I got to be Hyundai's National Youth Ambassador for Hope on Wheels 2008–2009.

ERIN: Cancer was a paradigm shift for Sammy. She realized there's a dark side to life and bad things can happen to you. All kids get that growing up, but she got it a lot faster than her peers.

> *Cancer doesn't just happen to you. It happens to the whole family.*

I worried, what did I do wrong? I said to God, "Why are you punishing my daughter for this? She didn't do anything, so what did I do?" But I see now why we're here—Sammy is inspirational. I believe that it is God's will that she be a torchbearer for other cancer survivors, for the other children. For the parents whose children didn't make it and who can't get up to talk, it's my job to tell their story. I gladly take on this role of activist. I speak for all those parents who can't speak about it or have lost the struggle. I have been mentoring at CHOC (Children's Hospital of Orange County) to help parents through this ordeal.

With this realization, I now know that God doesn't make these things happen. It's a matter of nature. God is here to help us through it.

We don't take anything for granted. Every day we are thankful for all of it. When I see her every day and get to love her or be annoyed by her, I am thankful for all of it. Even when she's a grouch, I'm thankful she's here to be a grouch.

SAMANTHA: Does that mean I'm allowed to be grouchy more often?

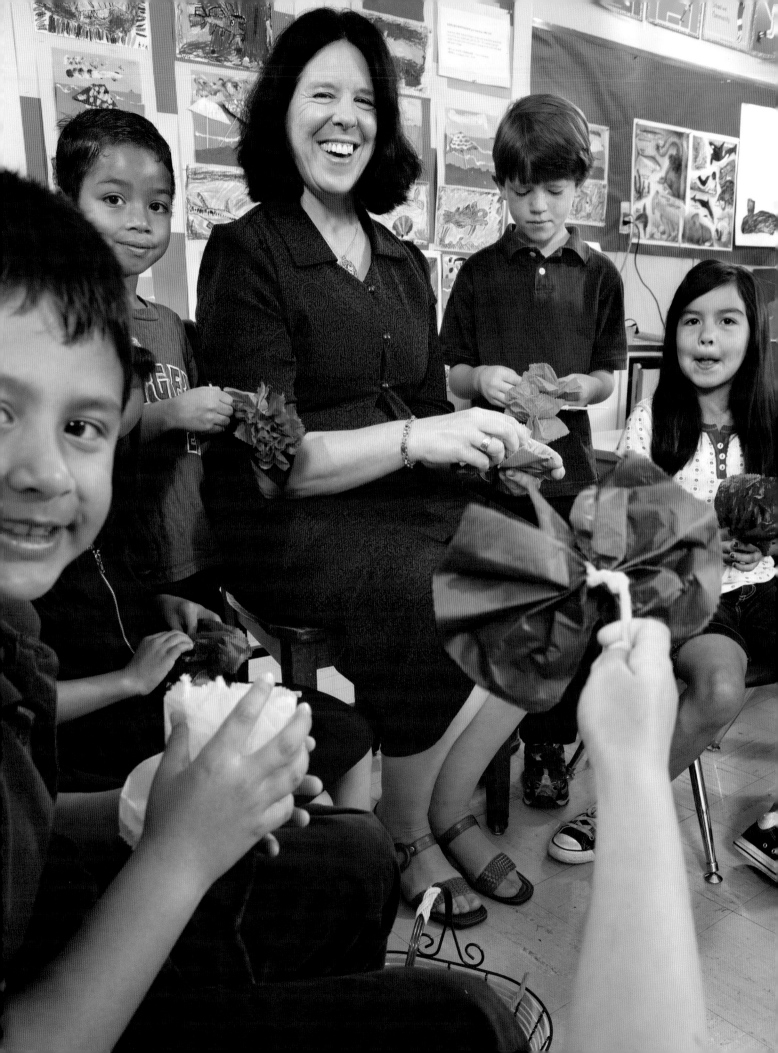

Shari Shapiro

Elementary Public School Teacher
Age at diagnosis, 49
Uterine sarcoma, 2001

Growing up, my routine annual checkups were always just that. Routine. More of a "hi" and "bye." In 2001 it was a longer conversation; I was diagnosed with uterine sarcoma.

The main memory I have of the months after that "sentence" is not of the medication or the side effects or the pain, but of my family's strong support. With their encouragement and my doctor's professional advice, I had two surgeries, underwent radiation, and eventually got through it.

I did initially have a few nights of crying, but I made a conscious decision to not let negativity overcome my even stronger determination for survival. My experience both in and out of the hospital opened my eyes to how blessed I was to have been diagnosed early. I tell all my women friends to get regular checkups. If I had waited just three or four more weeks, I wouldn't be healthy today.

> *I made a conscious decision to not let negativity overcome my even stronger determination for survival.*

After several months, I went back to teaching first graders at my elementary school, a job I have enjoyed for more than thirty years. I teach children to lead healthy lives, as well as reading, writing, and math. I emphasize being kind to one another and the importance of cooperation and teamwork. From my experiences I carry the lessons of compassion, sensitivity, and perseverance into every lesson plan I bring to the classroom.

I start every morning with the children singing "Row, Row, Row Your Boat!" This tradition is a reminder to me that even when the tides get rough, with supportive crew members and a focus on your goals, you will keep rowing gently along.

My husband, Lenny, is such a devoted husband. When I was sick, he gave me a little bell and pretended to be my butler.

Life for me now is all about the details. When I go to a concert, I concentrate on each instrument. And when I'm on the freeway going to work at 5:30 in the morning, instead of fretting about all the traffic, I watch the sun rise and listen to music.

P.S. When this book comes out, all the other teachers will finally know why my class was singing "Row, Row, Row Your Boat" at 8:00 every morning.

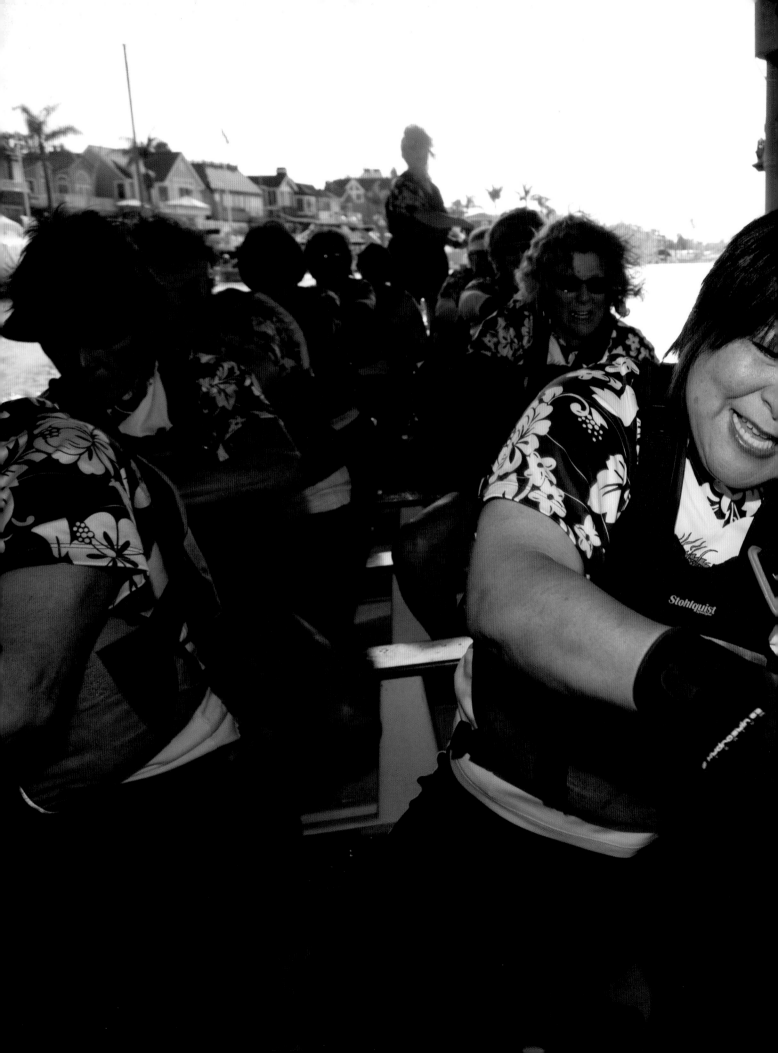

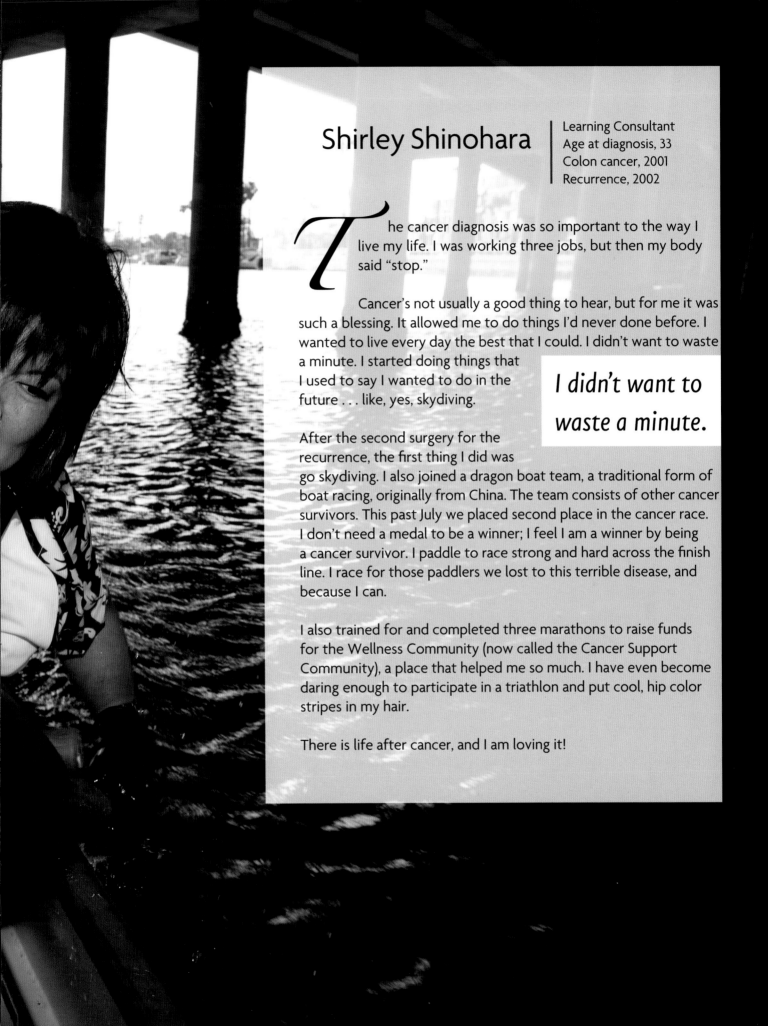

Shirley Shinohara

Learning Consultant
Age at diagnosis, 33
Colon cancer, 2001
Recurrence, 2002

The cancer diagnosis was so important to the way I live my life. I was working three jobs, but then my body said "stop."

Cancer's not usually a good thing to hear, but for me it was such a blessing. It allowed me to do things I'd never done before. I wanted to live every day the best that I could. I didn't want to waste a minute. I started doing things that I used to say I wanted to do in the future . . . like, yes, skydiving.

I didn't want to waste a minute.

After the second surgery for the recurrence, the first thing I did was go skydiving. I also joined a dragon boat team, a traditional form of boat racing, originally from China. The team consists of other cancer survivors. This past July we placed second place in the cancer race. I don't need a medal to be a winner; I feel I am a winner by being a cancer survivor. I paddle to race strong and hard across the finish line. I race for those paddlers we lost to this terrible disease, and because I can.

I also trained for and completed three marathons to raise funds for the Wellness Community (now called the Cancer Support Community), a place that helped me so much. I have even become daring enough to participate in a triathlon and put cool, hip color stripes in my hair.

There is life after cancer, and I am loving it!

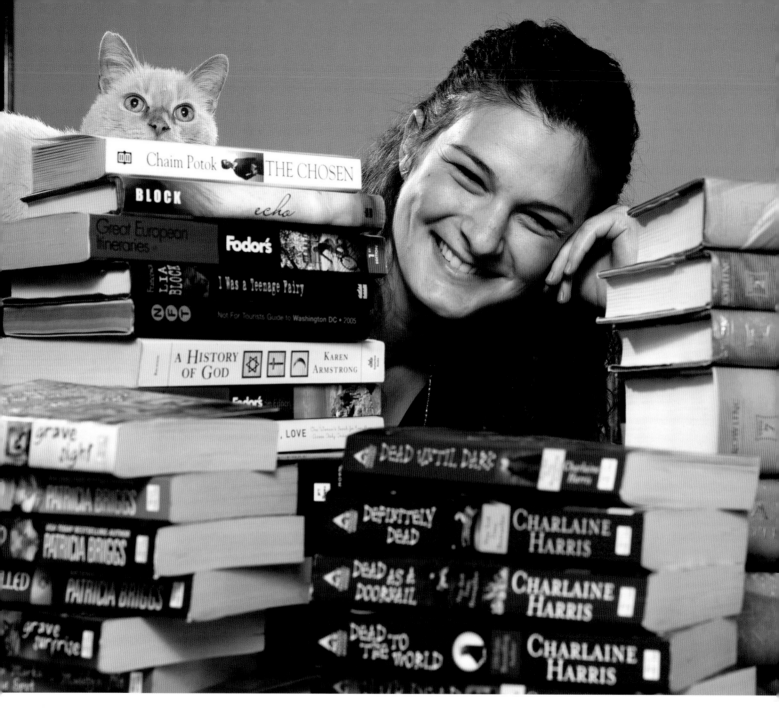

Life is so precious, and the pain that it can bring is a small price to pay for the joy of experiencing it.

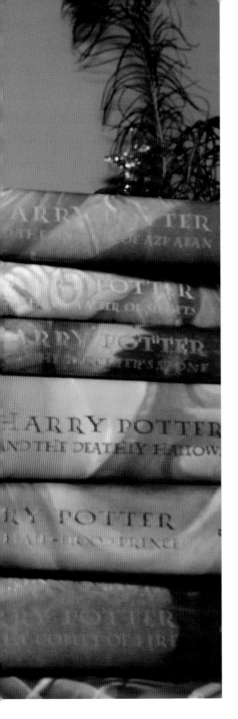

Shoshana Silver

Immigration Attorney
Age at diagnosis, 16
Synovial cell sarcoma, 1999

Cancer is something that happens to other people.

When I got my diagnosis, I locked myself in the bathroom and talked to God. I told Him, "I know you're God, and I'm not. Maybe I'm supposed to die, but I want you to know that I'm not ready yet."

Suddenly, all the small things in life were just bullshit. They didn't mean anything. It seemed like all of a sudden I knew what was true and what wasn't.

Not a day goes by that I don't think about cancer. I wonder what will happen if it comes back. It is hard to believe that I could have died or that it might happen again. It feels like a betrayal that I can't even trust my own body. Then again, I have a sense of security because I've been in remission for fifteen years. Maybe I have the same chance as anyone else.

I no longer feel invincible like a lot of young people do. I ask my friends who are smokers, "Why do you think it won't happen to you? You went through it with me." I hope they don't have to learn their vulnerability or harsh realities. Everyone deserves to hold on to innocence for as long as possible.

> *I no longer feel invincible like a lot of young people do.*

I now appreciate what I have and all the moments in my life. I love the little things, like looking up at the stars or watching the ocean. I feel happy and alive when I'm at family dinners or reading the next popular fiction in a series. I love fooling around with my crazy pets or going out dancing with friends. I go with my family every Friday night to the diner around the corner. It's a nice treat at the end of the week.

I have normal worries, which is a sign that my life is now normal. I appreciate what I have, and cherish every moment, even the bad ones. Life is so precious, and the pain that it can bring is a small price to pay for the joy of experiencing it. The joy of simply living.

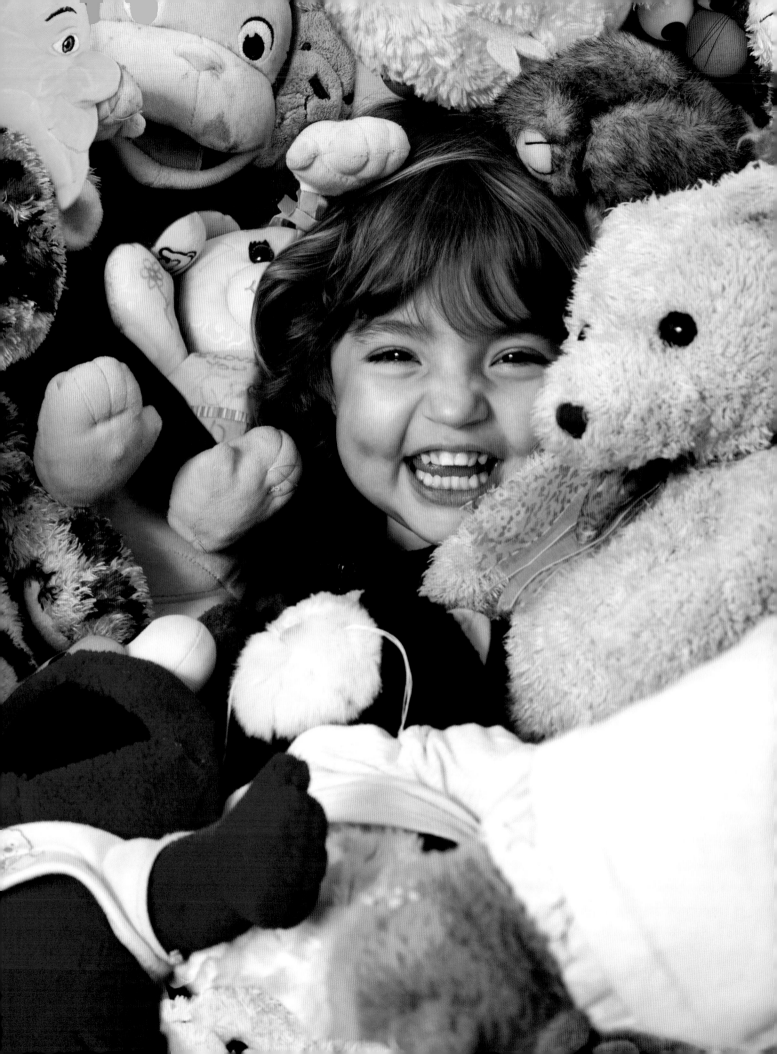

Sophia Colby

Age at diagnosis, 15 Months
Hemophagocytic lymphohistiocytosis
(HLH), 2005

SOPHIA'S FATHER, PATRICK: Sophia's disease is often diagnosed posthumously. It's often too late because testing takes too long. She was only a week and a half away from that point of no return. No one still knows how she survived. We were on a camping trip and had to see a doctor, who was able to diagnose her. We think of that camping trip as some sort of divine intervention.

Many things quickly changed. Right away we learned the importance of relationships with family and friends. As a male, my natural instinct was to close the doors and take care of my family. I now know that doesn't work. The offers of help started rolling in. We had no idea what we were in for, but when we finally said yes to help, the walls blew down and we realized the goodness of people. This allowed more people to be empowered to help.

There is nothing but good people out there. If we all would take off our daily blinders and open our eyes, we'd see a very positive and giving world. Unfortunately, a lot of people have to go through something horrible to see that.

Even though I could lose her tomorrow, I've already learned that life is joyful and empowering. Every day is fun. Even the difficult days have lessons to be learned. Sophia proved that.

> *There is nothing but good people out there.*

She was such a little social butterfly. She would knock on other patients' doors, even the depressed teenagers, and get them to come out and play. She was always happy, bouncing around, coloring, and dragging her IV pole around with her. One day the doctor looked at the nurse and asked, "Are you sure we're giving this kid chemo?"

SOPHIA'S MOTHER, BRIDGET: In 2009 we found out Sophie does not make B cells, the ones responsible for antibodies. The doctors don't know why, but she will need to have infusions every three weeks for the rest of her life to artificially boost her immune system.

Sophia is now ten years old and just started the fifth grade at a new school. We changed from private to public school to help her with some learning issues. She is making new friends and enjoys going to a school without uniforms.

She has a major purpose. We don't know what it is, but we think she's already doing it. During a terrible episode, when they were trying to restart her heart in the hospital, I looked up and saw all of the families of the other children outside her room cheering her on. I said to God, "How can you give her this special gift to bring so many people together and then take it away from all of them?"

Life is about moments. We have started to live day-by-day, hour-by-hour, and sometimes second-by-second. And when you sit there with those seconds seemingly so long, you realize how many of them you have.

> *Life is about moments.*

We have the luxury of seeing so many little gifts that other people don't see. The smell of my daughter's hair in the morning is one such gift. My favorite daily gift is getting to snuggle in the morning.

There is a constant reminder that she's borrowed. She's not ours.

Spencer Shiffman

Internet Salesman, Cancer Fund-Raiser
Age at first diagnosis, 25
Testicular cancer, 1986 and 1989
Peritoneal mesothelioma, 1994–2002

*E*very step of my cancer story is pretty miraculous. I never abused my body. I never drank, smoked, or did drugs. I never even had a hangnail. I was in the Little League World Series, was a quarterback in football, and have played golf since I was twelve. At twenty-four I ran the New York City Marathon. A few weeks after the race, I joked to a girl that I thought I was bloated and having my period. Soon after that, we started dating. She was a nurse and discovered my first testicular cancer.

Four days later, I had surgery. They told me I was fine and that I never again had to worry. Six weeks after the surgery, I ran a half marathon. Three years later, we were thinking about marriage, and she told me to find out what kind of live sperm I could produce with one testicle. During that visit, they discovered three more tumors on the remaining testicle. I banked sperm for ten days and then did my second surgery to remove my remaining testicle.

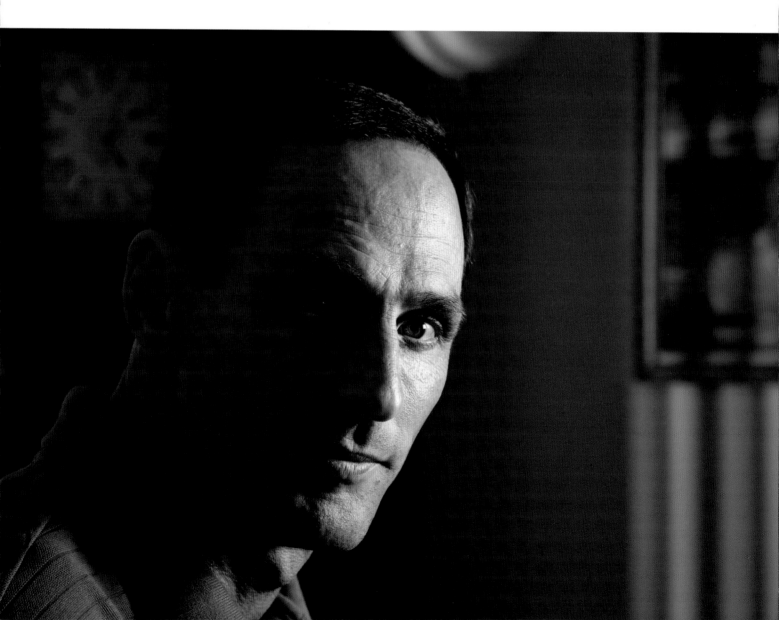

One month away from being five years in remission, I was playing golf. I thought my appendix burst, but, once again, it was cancer, peritoneal mesothelioma. This time doctors said there was no cure. I flew to Austin every week for nine months for experimental treatment, but without success. I went back to conventional chemotherapy, but that didn't work either.

After that I went to Houston for another experimental treatment. I sat in that office for four hours each time, waiting for my appointment and looking at the children with brain cancer. The kids played with toys, but the parents had so much sadness. I told my mom, "If I live, I want to give back. It's not fair that these kids have to live with this and not even know it's not normal." After nine months of that treatment, the tumors grew so big I looked pregnant. After a fourteen-pound tumor was removed, I went on hospice care. I still refused to believe I was going to die.

For the next three years I was addicted to pain medications, including dilaudid and morphine. I got a blood transfusion every month. The doctors said I couldn't live through a surgery, but I told them I wanted to sign my life away and do it. Miraculously, I made it.

A few months later I got pneumonia and told my parents to just let me die. I couldn't fight any longer. My friend Joe Pesci heard that, came and jumped into my hospital bed, and said, "No one is going to let you die, so forget about it!" I now call him my muse. After that, I never looked back. My survival proved that you can't give up. My motto is "Never give up, there's always *hope*."

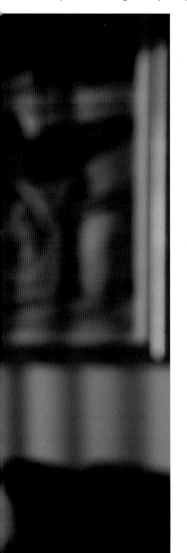

For the next four years, I held annual golf tournaments and raised money for pediatric cancer research. I also produced celebrity-filled fund-raisers for Cure Search and City of Hope Hospital.

I eventually had to concentrate on my well-being and move away from my life of cancer. After ten years, I got back into the real world and started to deal with love, emotions, and responsibilities. In 2006 at forty-five, I began discovering who I am for the first time. I started to live and now look forward to so many things. It's amazing.

I'm fifty-two now. I play golf two to three times a week and work hard in my business. Just like my license plate says "CNCRWNR," I'm a "Cancer Winner."

Just like my license plate says "CNCRWNR," I'm a "Cancer Winner."

Stefanie LaRue

Model and Organizational Spokesperson,
Speaker, Realtor
Age at diagnosis, 30
Stage 4 Metastatic breast cancer, 2005
Recurrences 2008, 2010, 2013

When doctors told me I had nine months to live in 2005, I immediately went out and got two tattoos: one with the predicted date of death and a second with the Phoenix rising from the ashes. From that day on, I became determined to enjoy every moment of life.

Three prior physicians had misdiagnosed me. They said that young pretty girls don't get breast cancer. I screamed, cried, cussed, begged, and demanded to finally get the biopsy. By that point, the cancer had already metastasized to my spine. Stage 4. Nine months. Good luck.

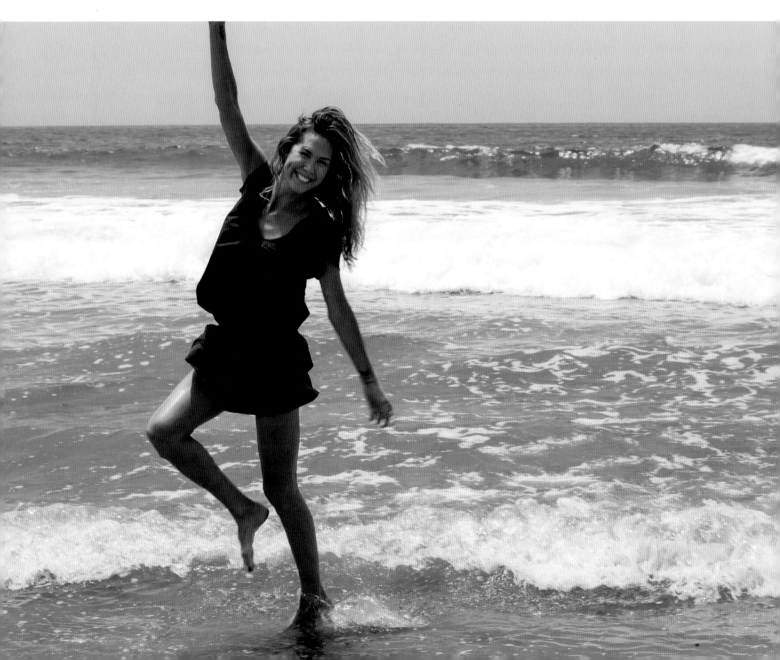

Some people don't allow cancer to change them. They get caught in the negativity and can't do what it takes to save their lives. You have to learn to pick up the pieces when they all fall apart. I learned that I needed to live life exactly as it was being handed to me. I needed to be present in Stage 4 because there is no Stage 5.

I received the most rigorous chemotherapy possible. It's so toxic that they don't even give it any more. I was quarantined with zero white blood cells and almost died. But I survived and turned to good, healthy food and supplements, combined with a new power of mind, body, and soul to boost my immune system. You have to stay hungry to allow your spirit to grow. I came out of that hospital starving.

After two years of physical therapy, I went through the darkest period of my life. I lost my disability income, and my family started crumbling around me.

I went back into the workforce, but I struggled and often resorted to hiding. The stressful environment didn't allow me to take care of myself in a way that I knew was vital. I knew what was happening, and, sure enough, the first recurrence came in 2008, less than three years after my first treatments. The beast was back. I soon began targeted radiation.

I tried to keep working, but recurrence number two, a tumor on the top of my left hip, came along in 2010. I had more radiation, and I was clean again until 2013. This time, the shit hit the fan: multiple tumors reared their ugly heads. The doctors encouraged surgery and removed my thymus, the gland that produces t-cells. They then offered me all new options for chemo again.

I wanted to explore other options, so I reached out to my community and to social media. I read, researched, and received assistance with the inundation of information and eventually discovered hemp oil. It is now saving my life. I ingest one gram of oil per day, high in CBD (medicinal value) and low in THC ("stoner" effect). This is my personal journey, and it's working for me. Every month my tumor markers are lower.

Cancer has changed everything for me. At my first breast cancer conference, the Young Survivors Coalition Conference, I was confronted with many women my age who were similarly imperiled. We all shared and cried together but that only put a big fear bubble in my head. For many of us, losing our fertility was the most devastating part.

I'm still trying to learn how to feel normal again in society. I'm a people person, and I like to get out and meet and explore. That's essential for my healing process. I am still choosing to live life despite the fear, family deaths, and uncertainty.

I'm in a new relationship with a woman I met a year and a half ago. I've never felt a deep connection like this before in my life.

I have learned from cancer that life should be about making memories, helping others, and nourishing our souls. I wish that all survivors could learn to breathe in that breath of fresh air. I am now surrounding myself with laughter, friends, and peaceful healing.

That's my brand. That's me. Live Organic; Live Orgasmic. I wonder if that would fit on a tattoo?

> *I have learned from cancer that life should be about making memories, helping others, and nourishing our souls.*

Stephen Macht

Actor, Jewish Chaplain
Age at diagnosis, 68
Prostate cancer, 2010

I feel very lucky. When my doctor discovered elevated PSA levels, he sent me to a urologist because of my family history of cancer. That specialist said he felt a small node but not to worry and to come back in three weeks. My internist insisted that I go back right away. A day and a half later, I was back in the urologist's office. He took twenty-one biopsies and confirmed an aggressive prostate cancer.

Because I have a mild case of colitis, radiation was out of the question. I had one choice: surgery. I chose the surgeon who said, "Let's try to save everything" instead of the one who subscribed to the "Let's take out everything just to be safe" theory. Six weeks later, after robotic surgery, my surgeon announced, "We got the bastard."

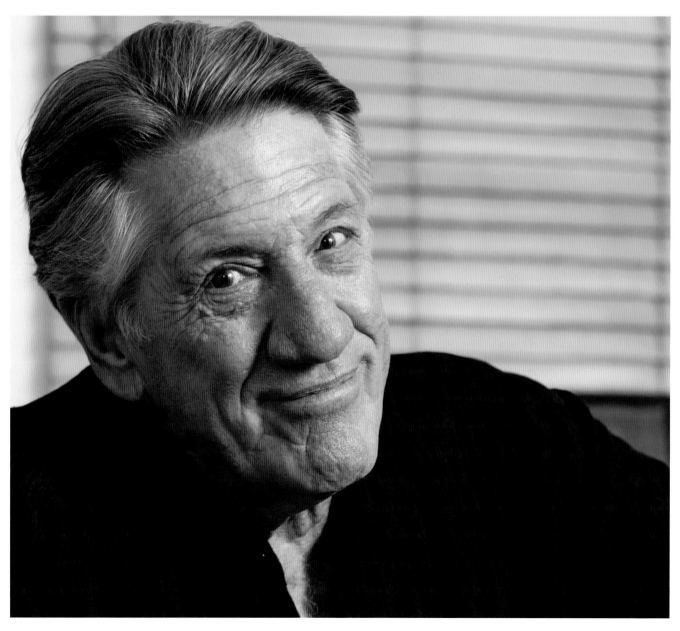

Four years later, the cancer is still undetectable.

Those are the physical facts, but a lot of emotional stuff comes along with it.

My father died of cancer at age forty-four when I was nine years old. My wife, Suzanne, and I were married in the cancer ward when my mom was dying, at age fifty-six. I never thought I would live past forty-five years old. These are the dark assumptions that little boys make.

When my father died, my mother told me that he was "in a better place." But I looked at his open coffin and saw his balding head and thought two things: *I'm never going to die like you and I'm going to bring you back.* Since then, I have lived my life running away from this fear of dying.

To cover those fears, I decided that nothing was going to stop me. "If I couldn't do something by myself, I wouldn't do it." This was my operating principle. But I began to realize, if one does this, always acting in your own best interests, you cut out 85 to 90 percent of the world. Plus you tend to have anger issues with people who don't live up to your expectations.

As I grew older and started to study acting, I had two great teachers: an acting coach and a rabbi. The rabbi put his finger on my anger problems. "You've never mourned. Why don't you do it now."

He gave me a mantra and told me to recite it morning, noon and night. "Your father will not save you. Your mother will not save you. Neither will your god." At last, with a lot of tears and sadness, I began to look at and mourn all of those losses and all the mistakes I made, all the misplaced anger. I started to accept responsibility for my own life without blaming others.

That mantra became a springboard for my study as a Jewish chaplain.

Part of my learning has been *Teshuvah*, which means returning to the best of who you are meant to be. In order to return to the best of who you are, you must discover the mistakes that you make. You have to take an accounting of your soul.

> The cancer has reinforced and strengthened a path that I was already on.

It's still a process. A few days ago, somebody cut in front of me, and road rage and cursing came right out. My wife was prepared. She held up a cardboard cutout with the face of my rabbi pasted to a chopstick. "If he was in the car, you would be ashamed. You would never behave like that. Plus, it's not very Chaplinesque." We began laughing so hard that I had to park the car. Now I realize that I've got to be my own restraining image. I can't wait for my wife to put the lollipop up. That's part of the return. To let it go instead of cursing that son of a bitch.

Cancer was also part of the change, part of my returning. It got me to look at whatever life I've got left and ask myself, "How are you going to use it?" Are you still going to make choices about not getting your father back? About not dying? Or are you going to spend your life in service of others and help sustain life?

The cancer has reinforced and strengthened a path that I was already on.

To enjoy my life and share it. And to make positive contributions to the world whenever I can without denigrating anyone and without expecting anything.

Just last week when my son, Gabriel, directed me as an actor, he looked at me and said, "Take away all the makeup and just be quiet. Be yourself. You're really powerful when you're quiet. Don't garnish it." What an amazing experience to be told something like that by your son. He was helping me to return to the best of myself.

It's awe-inspiring when I think about it.

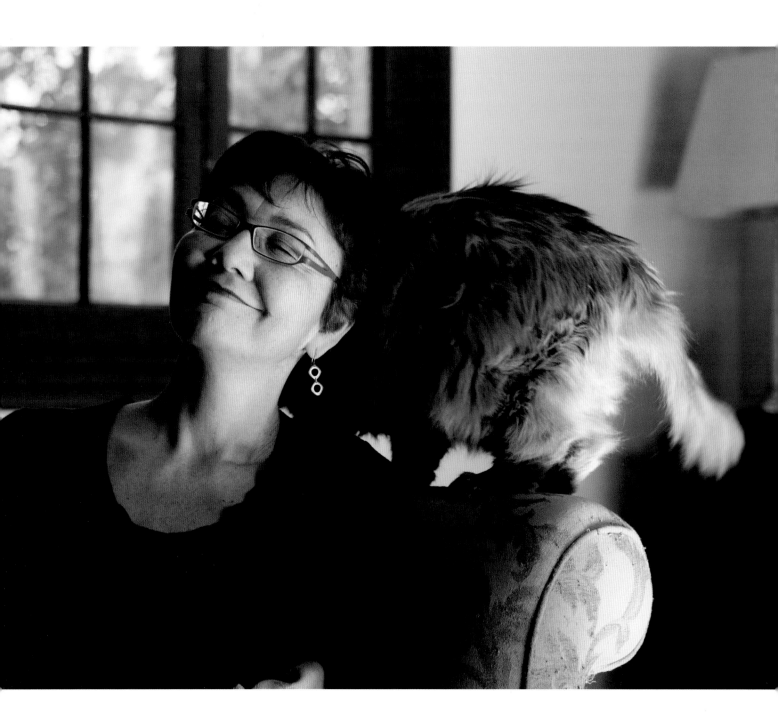

Susan Carrier

Writer, Editor, Marketing Consultant
Age at diagnosis, 53
Blastic mantle cell, non-Hodgkin's lymphoma, 2007

*I*t's now been more than seven years since I discovered that my droopy-looking right eye wasn't just an annoying reminder of my advancing years. After playing a round of "stump the ophthalmologists," I went to an optical surgeon for a biopsy. I was stunned to find out that lump under my eyelid was a cancerous tumor from a rare blood cancer.

These days I rarely think or talk about cancer, a far cry from the early days when every waking thought revolved around the disease. When I wasn't obsessively studying the diagnosis or the treatment, I was posting daily updates on my blog, *Cancer Banter*.

Just when I thought I couldn't be more obsessed, a doctor from a prestigious hospital informed me and a room full of patients that our particular type of MCL always comes back. ("It's not *if* you will relapse, but *when*.") After hearing this encouraging news, I spent a weekend holed up in my bedroom, analyzing spreadsheets and attempting to predict the day of my death.

Given the odds, I was relieved to receive a stem cell transplant with my own harvested stem cells. The worst hours were the thirty-six hours post transplant, when I was curled up in a fetal position, weak and nauseous. But the harsh treatments did the trick, and I went into and stayed in remission.

One of the things I have learned from being a patient and being a parent is that we have no control. We think we have control over what's going on in our lives, but it is all an illusion. We only have control over our attitudes.

A few months ago at a party, an old friend gushed, "You must wake up every morning so grateful to be alive." I hesitated because I knew what she wanted to hear and I didn't want to disappoint her. But then I looked her straight in the eye and laughed, "Oh, hell no." We both wondered what had happened to my initial post-remission euphoria.

And what had happened to my fearless, new, chance-taking approach to life that I bragged about shortly after my stem cell transplant? As it turns out, the attitude of gratitude and the willingness to leave our comfort zones are both muscles that I need to flex and work every single day.

> *The attitude of gratitude and the willingness to leave our comfort zones are both muscles that I need to flex and work every single day.*

Susan Love

Founder and Chief Visionary Officer,
Dr. Susan Love Research Foundation;
Author of *Dr. Susan Love's Breast Book*
Age at diagnosis, 64
Acute myeloid leukemia (AML), 2012

*T*he only difference between a researcher and a patient is a diagnosis.

The diagnosis was a total shock. It makes no difference if you're a physician, it still scares you . . . scares you to death. As a physician, I started a foundation focused on finding the cause and prevention of breast cancer, and all of a sudden, on June 8, 2012, I was the patient. I had no obvious symptoms

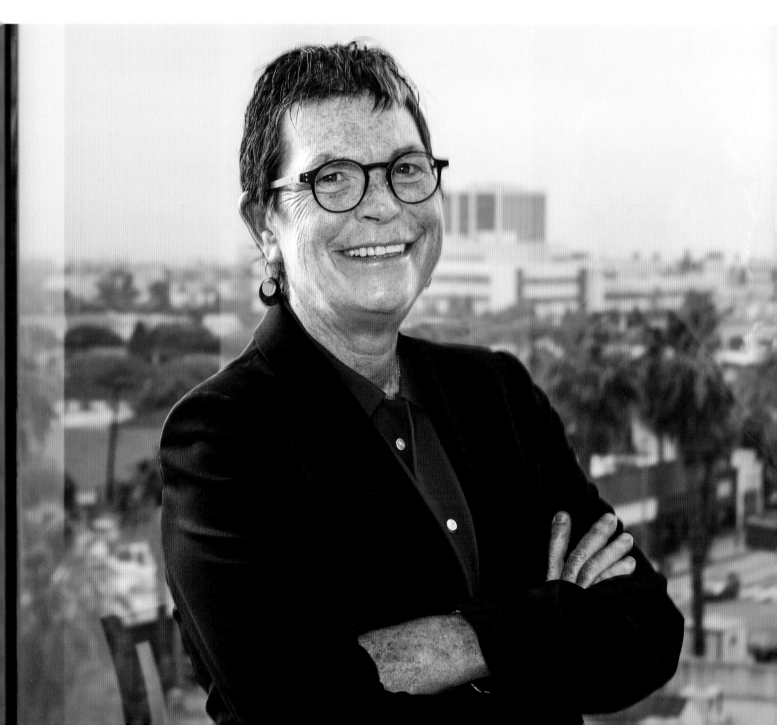

and learned of my disease only after a checkup and routine blood work. It was really out of the blue. I was feeling fine. I had run five miles the day before.

In some ways it would have been less shocking if it were breast cancer, but getting leukemia was a world I didn't know.

Because I had no symptoms, I had a little time to get a second opinion and decide on a medical team. I chose City of Hope Hospital because of its extensive experience in bone marrow transplants. I was somewhat chagrined to find out that at age sixty-four I was considered among the "elderly" patients for this type of leukemia.

There is no surgery for leukemia, so I immediately began chemotherapy. After seven weeks in the hospital, my blood counts had still not come back to normal, so I was scheduled for a bone marrow transplant. I was blessed that my youngest sister, Elizabeth, was a donor match. The transplant procedure is pretty rigorous because it involves killing off your own bone marrow with chemotherapy and then replacing it with your donor's cells. It's interesting to me that your blood type changes to that of your donor's and all your allergies disappear.

The only difference between a researcher and a patient is a diagnosis.

My wife, Helen, and my daughter, Katie, were there for me around the clock. Between them and my wonderful siblings, I was never alone in the hospital. I realized that you need doctors to take care of you, but your family is there to be your advocates.

My life has been a big adventure. I am the oldest of five children and was raised Catholic. I spent six months as a nun, and then I "kicked the habit." Now I have been with my wife for thirty years and have a beautiful twenty-five-year-old daughter. My sudden illness made me grateful that we hadn't postponed exploring our bucket list. I have focused on work I find challenging and satisfying and explored the world, and as of now my bone marrow is clean and I'm feeling stronger. My life is getting back on track.

The experience of being a patient has brought home to me the amount of temporary and permanent side effects caused by our treatments. I think we have to go beyond finding the cure, with all of its collateral damage, to finding the cause. We have to stop people from getting cancer in the first place.

Having cancer myself has given me a new sense of urgency. We have a limited number of days in our lives—you become more aware of that—and if I'm going to spend them coming to work, then I'm not going to be just diddling around.

I often tell my daughter that whether it's changing the world or having a good time, we should not put off what we think we should do. You never know when you will be caught up short with a serious disease. We are all patients eventually.

That's why I drink the expensive wine now.

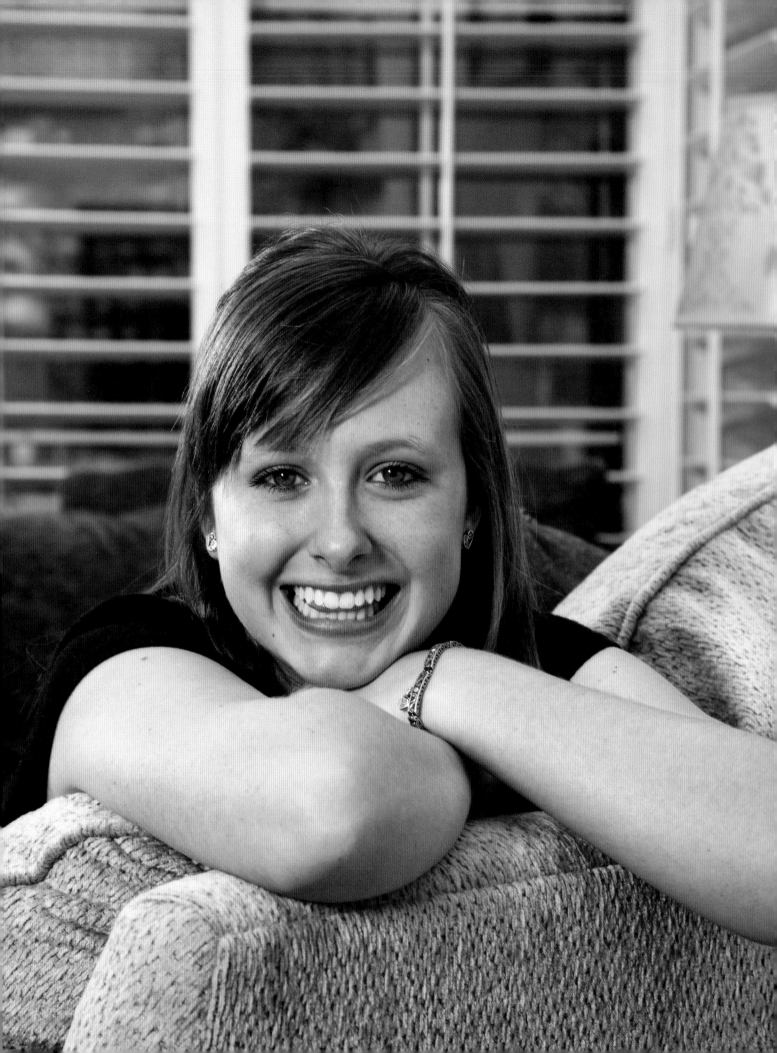

Tara Hussey

Age at diagnosis, 14
Acute lymphoblastic
leukemia (ALL), 2005

TARA: Out of everyone I know, I was the right person to get cancer because I wouldn't give up and wouldn't let it get me down.

From the very beginning, I told my family, "We'll get through this. We need to have a positive attitude." And then everyone jumped in. My friends were such a huge support. They had a crepe sale at school and bought me a laptop so I could communicate with all of them. Entire classes made cards for me. They even sold wristbands that said TARA'S BUDDIES and raised over $25,000.

You have to have faith in God that He put this in your life to make you stronger, not as something to beat you down or stop you. In my mind, I wasn't allowed to give up. Instead, I knew this would change my path in life and how I would view life from then on.

Before cancer, I wanted to be a teacher, but now I want to be a pediatric oncology nurse. It's odd, but now cancer is my passion. I love talking about it, helping people, and I even do a lot of public speaking for The Leukemia & Lymphoma Society. I just love talking about cancer. I'm excited to tell people what I went through, and if they feel shy in asking me questions, I assure them I will tell them anything they want to ask.

I had epilepsy until I was ten, and then just before cancer, I had scoliosis. So I just keep learning and growing. But I have to tell you, if someone tells me about a blood drive, I say, "Trust me. You don't want my blood."

My friends were such a huge support. They had a crepe sale at school and bought me a laptop so I could communicate with all of them.

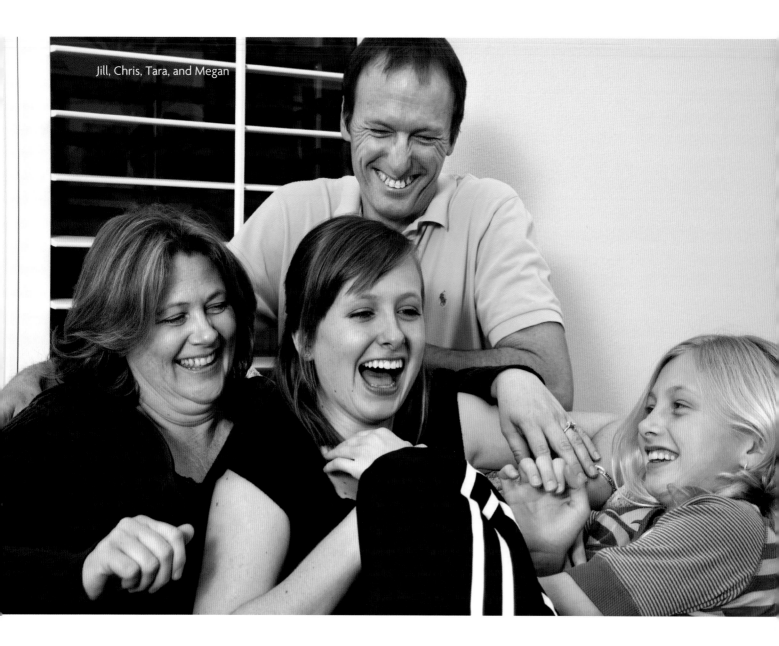

Jill, Chris, Tara, and Megan

CHRIS, TARA'S FATHER: In the beginning, a friend at church told us, "You've been given a path. You can't go around it, over it, or under it. You have to walk through it." And we did, with faith as a family. And we had fun. We were the ones laughing and having fun on the floor at the hospital.

JILL, TARA'S MOTHER: Her friends are dealing with sex, drugs, and alcohol, but she is already talking about her future. She tells them, "Oh, I've already done all the drugs. I'm done." From a parent's perspective, no child should have to grow up so quickly, but grow up she did.

TARA: Like a normal teenager, before cancer I wanted to separate from my family, and now I can't get enough of them. I just want to stay home all the time.

Awarded :

(1)   The American Cancer Society's Youth Survivor Scholarship, 2008;

(2)   The Leukemia/Lymphoma Society's Honored Hero for "Light The Night" Walk, 2006

(3)   The Leukemia/Lymphoma Society's Honored Hero for "Pennies For Patients," 2007 & 2008

Like a normal teenager, before cancer I wanted to separate from my family, and now I can't get enough of them.

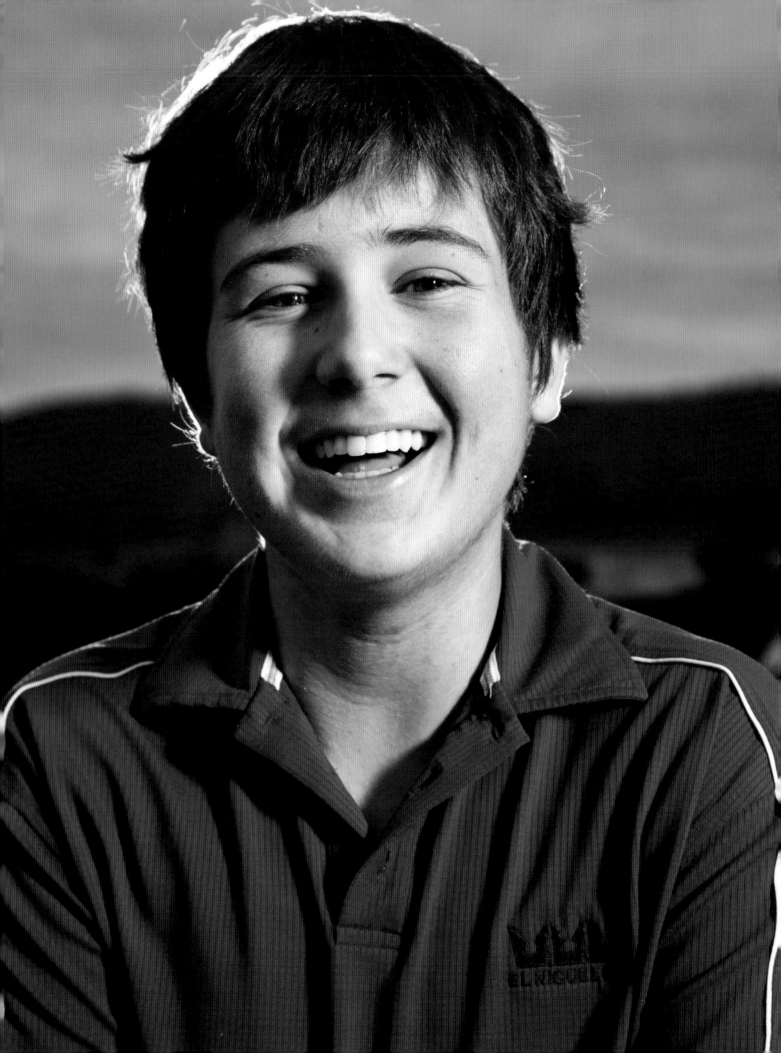

Taylor Carol

Age at diagnosis, 12
Acute lymphoblastic leukemia (ALL)
with Philadelphia chromosome, 2006

TAYLOR: It's hard to remember the first couple of months. I was in shock.

JIM, TAYLOR'S FATHER: Taylor is right. When you first find out the news, it's like being in a washing machine. You're just getting tumbled. You have to wake up every day and put one foot in front of the other. You have to let the day go where it's going to go.

He was diagnosed as terminal. It was a brutal, viscous, horrible treatment, and yet he led us in his own recovery. Never once did he complain or lose his faith. He showed a character that was amazing.

CYNTHIA, TAYLOR'S MOTHER: Doctors who were as brilliant as they were compassionate surrounded Taylor. We asked them for advice that might help us. These hard-core research scientists said they couldn't give exact statistics, but they could definitely tell us that kids who know the truth, are up for the battle, and are surrounded by love and a strong support system will always do better.

TAYLOR: My doctor said that getting well is 50 percent medicine and 50 percent mental. The people at the hospital knew that I liked to sing, so they brought in a musical therapist. I ended up getting to sing publicly with famous musicians and songwriters.

I've learned that disease can tear apart a family, but my experience has been a family that is stronger and closer.

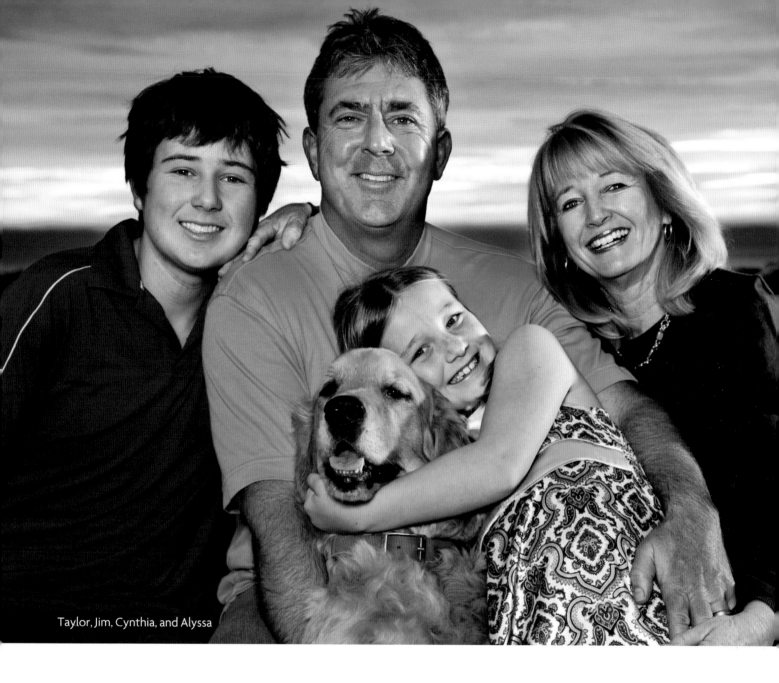

Taylor, Jim, Cynthia, and Alyssa

CYNTHIA: One of our most amazing moments was while Taylor was on stage singing a very emotional song called "Ordinary Miracles," and this beautiful twenty-seven-year-old, six-foot-five German guy came out and met him on stage. It was his bone marrow donor. We surprised Taylor and flew him in from Germany. They had never met.

TAYLOR: I've learned that disease can tear apart a family, but my experience has been a family that is stronger and closer. We were focused on healing and helping. They have really taught me what it means to be unselfish and give more than you receive. Even my little sister was such a trooper and sacrificed so much.

It's hard for me to say what I would have been if I hadn't gone through this, but I know for a fact that I'm a better person because of it. I believe that everything in life happens for a reason. The true purpose may not have arisen yet, but I can tell you that I am thankful for every day.

My notion of God is all the good in the world. When I pray, I close my eyes and see myself completely healthy. I try to see how I can improve and become closer to God. I've learned that the prayers that come true are the wishes that will truly make me a better person.

TAYLOR: It's been a long journey since 2006. I began traveling around the country to perform at fundraisers for sick children and pediatric cancer research. I've also sung or spoken at close to twenty fundraisers for Make-A-Wish Foundation. I performed the national anthem more than once at Clippers' and Angels' games. I feel like my illness and circumstances have helped me rise above and give hope to other people

I am now at Harvard University, and music is still my passion. I describe myself as a singer, a songwriter, and a lover of Life!

Taylor is a spokesperson for Beckstrand Cancer Foundation, Children's Hospital of Seattle, Jamie Moyer Foundation, Symphony Guild for Uncompensated Care, Hyundai Hope on Wheels, Hope Labs, Robert Woods Johnson Foundation, and Chordoma Foundation.

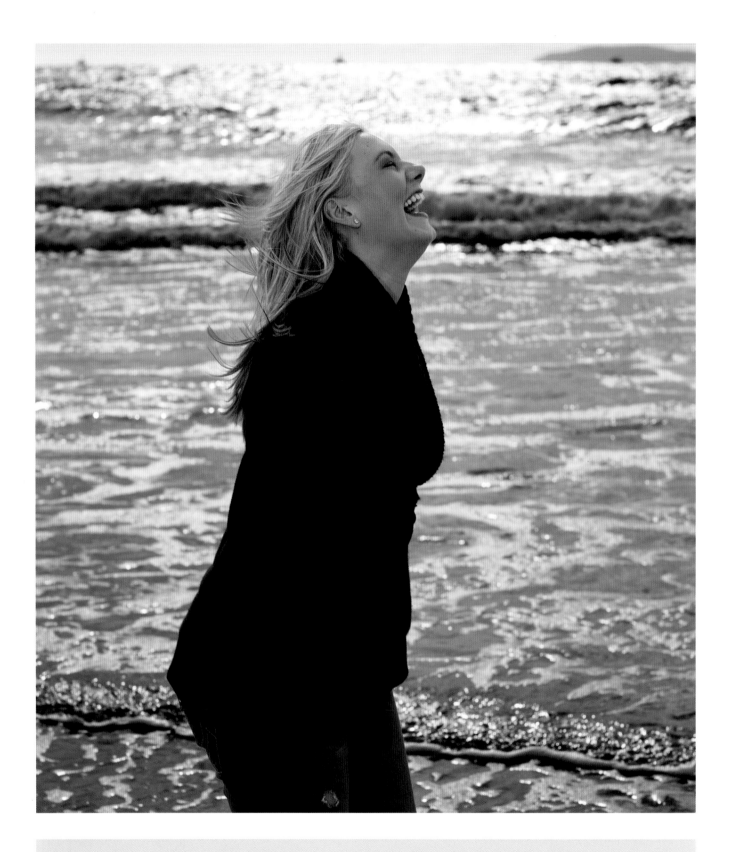

The self I came out of cancer with is much better than the self I had when I went in. If all I had to do was lose my hair and a piece of my arm, it was worth it.

Tiffany Graley

Accounting, Payroll
Age at diagnosis, 22
Ewing's sarcoma, 2004

I swam and played water polo my entire life, but one day a doctor looked at scans of my arm and told me that what he saw was life threatening. A tumor was growing so big and so fast, it was breaking the bone, and they needed to operate right away.

When I woke up from surgery, it felt like I had a bullet in my chest. I knew I had cancer, and I was so angry, I just wanted to strangle everyone in the room. I was twenty-two and had plans. I certainly wasn't prepared to start chemo the next day.

Life didn't seem fair. My parents had just gotten a divorce and my best friend had died in a car accident. Plus, my brother has autism and can't speak. I had just graduated from college and I was finally starting to get my life together. Cancer made it feel like it was all being ripped away; I felt helpless. After I left the hospital, I just stood in the parking lot screaming and crying.

My treatments were six hours a day, five days a week. When my hair started to fall out, a friend gave me a Mohawk and later shaved my head. During the next surgery, they removed four inches of my radius bone. For a year, I had no function in my arm, but I was lucky because not long ago, they would have cut off my arm.

One day in chemo I fainted. They told me it might be a tumor in my brain. I freaked out. A beautiful Asian girl came over and sat next to me. It was intimidating because I was bald and bloated, with no make-up, feeling like crap, and she was so beautiful. She put her arms around me and comforted me. That day I knew I had met an angel. From then on, through every treatment, we were always by each other's side. One morning I found out she had died. I wondered why God didn't take me because she was so good. He put her in my life to save my life and then took hers.

Once again, I was alone. I didn't know anyone else my age with cancer. Then I discovered "Planet Cancer," an online support group for young survivors just like me. I could heal and help others heal in this place. My angel had changed my life forever. I had a duty to teach what she had taught me: listen to others and not to my pain; be kind, not selfish. Everyone is battling something. I realized that I'm not a lone soldier.

I feel like it is such a blessing to be in this book. Not all cancer survivors can be famous, but we're all survivors and want to help as many others as we can. And I have to do twice as much because I'm now living for two of us.

Cancer gave me a new lease on life. I would never wish cancer on anyone, and it will probably always be the hardest thing I'll ever have to go through, but it made me alive in my faith. I don't take my life for granted now. You never know when it might be gone. The self I came out of cancer with is much better than the self I had when I went in. If all I had to do was lose my hair and a piece of my arm, it was worth it.

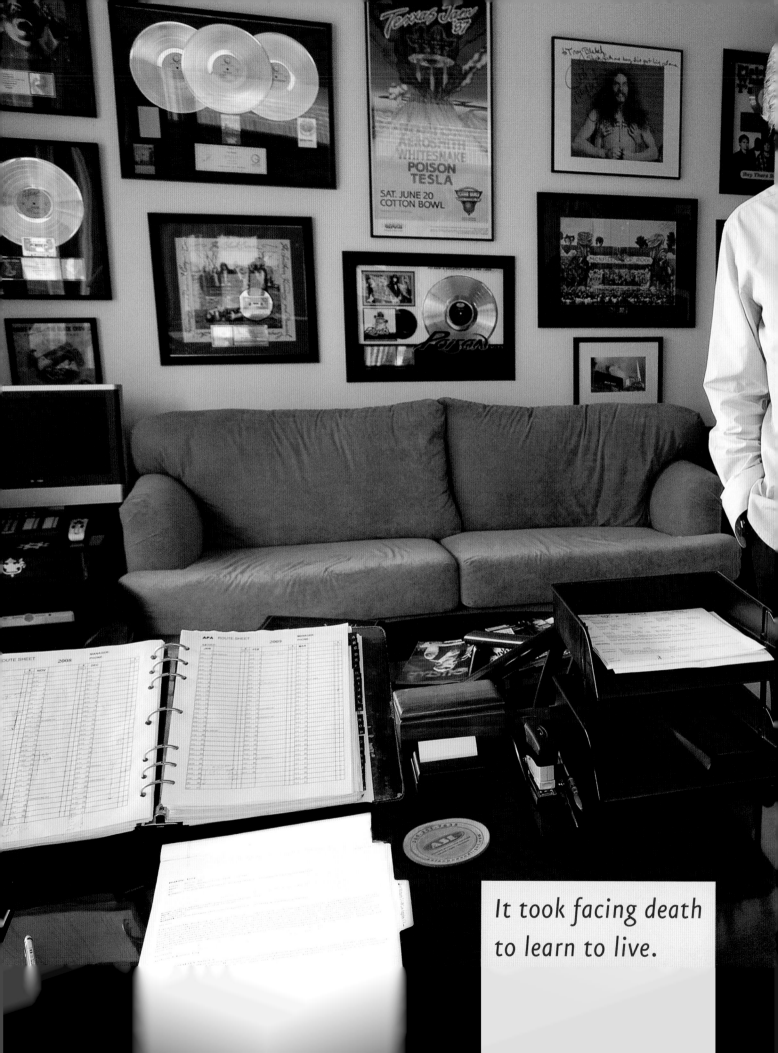

It took facing death
to learn to live.

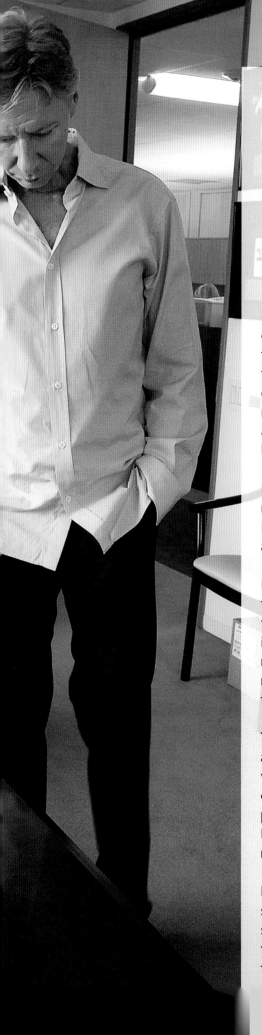

Troy Blakely

Talent Agent
Age at diagnosis, 44
Squamous cell carcinoma, 1994

When I was diagnosed, everyone said to me, "You're the healthiest person I know. You run marathons and eat brown rice all the time. How can *you* get cancer?" They didn't know the other side of me, the stress side.

I was suddenly challenged with the ultimate fear, losing my life. I started to think about all the things I might miss. It gave me determination to stay and to fight. After that, every occasion became special. I rarely talked about the negatives. They were there, but the best thing I could do was to have a positive attitude. I believe that if you sit around and mope, you will never heal. You have to fight the doubts, the fear, the anger, and all the things that creep in. The mind can do amazing things, both good and bad.

I remember lying awake at night thinking there was something inside of me that could kill me. It was part of me, and somehow I created it. So I owned it. I looked for control and I searched for answers. I constantly asked doctors, "How did I get this?" None of them could fill in that blank.

I'm the type of person who is always in control. While going through treatment, I felt incredibly helpless and at the mercy of the doctors. I listened to tapes that were created for cancer patients to visualize healing. I imagined my body attacking the cancer cells. It put me into a completely relaxed, hypnotic state. It gave me a way to be a participant in my treatment, and it kept me from feeling helpless. Instead, I was energized and felt much better.

Those months of treatments gave me a chance to focus on my life and examine my priorities. I was then able to return to my work without fear. I realized that I was damn good at my job and I wanted to continue with the career I had. Since then, my life—work and personal—has been amazing. In a very real sense, cancer rescued me. Instead of being afraid and insecure of who I was, I became who I really am.

I'm one of the most blessed people I know. What has happened to me since cancer—my career, becoming a partner at a major talent agency, seeing my son graduate high school and college and get married, and the birth of my grandson—I owe it all to the change I went through. It took facing death to learn to live.

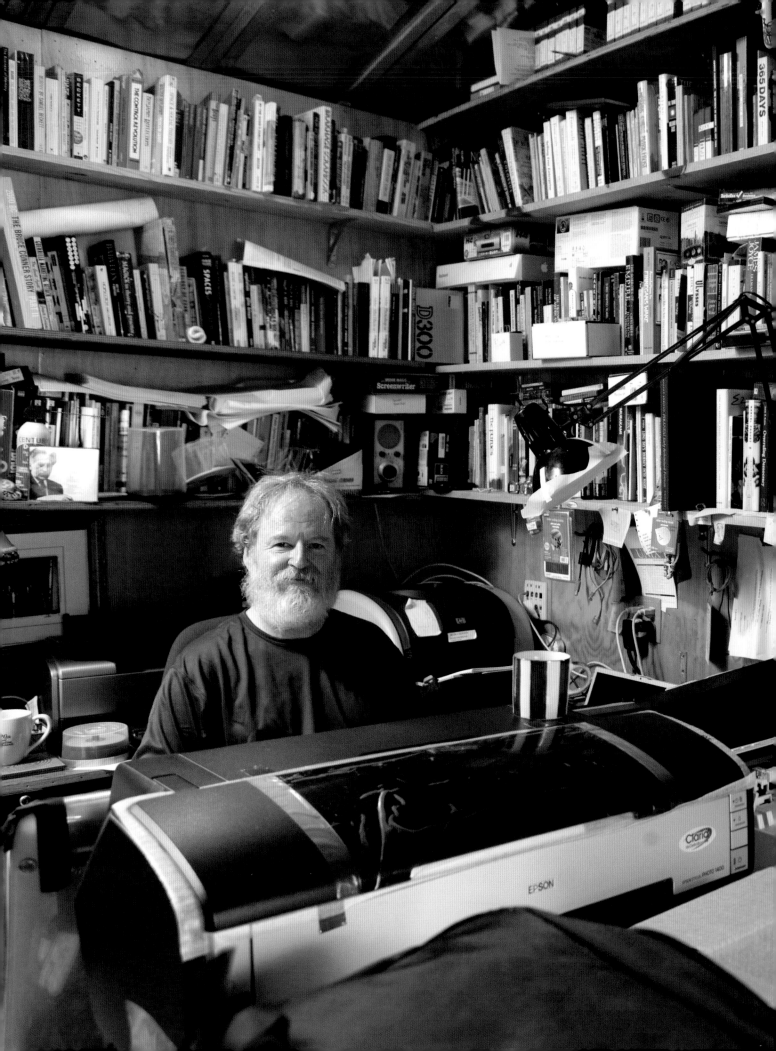

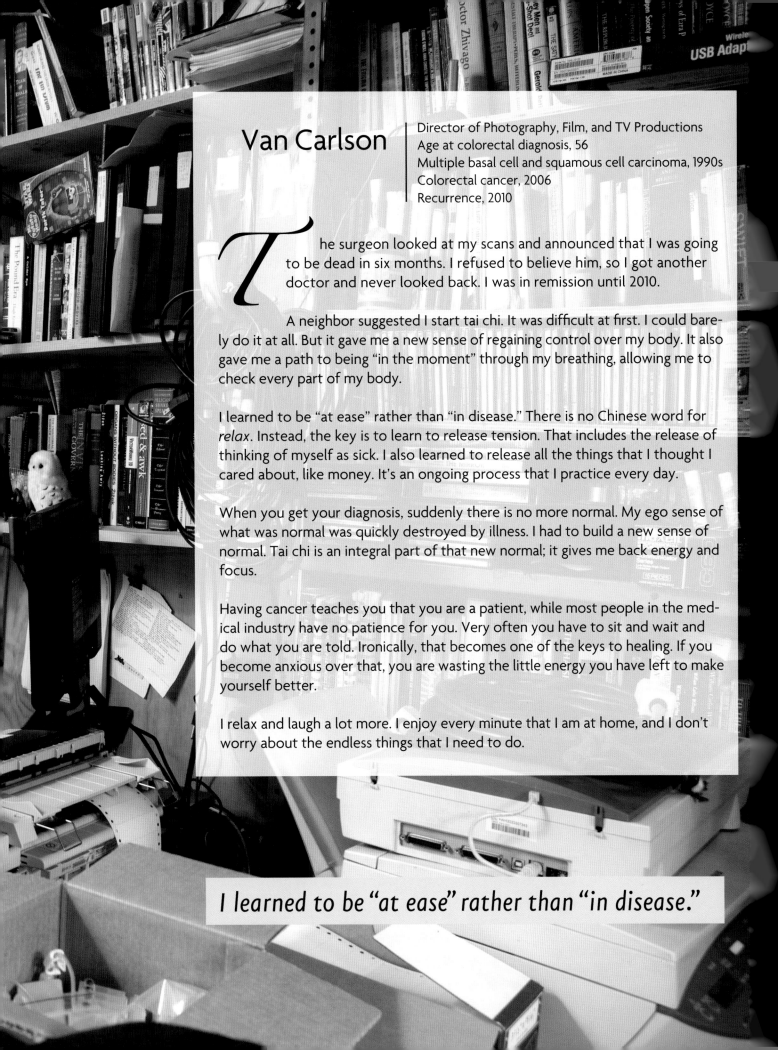

Van Carlson

Director of Photography, Film, and TV Productions
Age at colorectal diagnosis, 56
Multiple basal cell and squamous cell carcinoma, 1990s
Colorectal cancer, 2006
Recurrence, 2010

The surgeon looked at my scans and announced that I was going to be dead in six months. I refused to believe him, so I got another doctor and never looked back. I was in remission until 2010.

A neighbor suggested I start tai chi. It was difficult at first. I could barely do it at all. But it gave me a new sense of regaining control over my body. It also gave me a path to being "in the moment" through my breathing, allowing me to check every part of my body.

I learned to be "at ease" rather than "in disease." There is no Chinese word for *relax*. Instead, the key is to learn to release tension. That includes the release of thinking of myself as sick. I also learned to release all the things that I thought I cared about, like money. It's an ongoing process that I practice every day.

When you get your diagnosis, suddenly there is no more normal. My ego sense of what was normal was quickly destroyed by illness. I had to build a new sense of normal. Tai chi is an integral part of that new normal; it gives me back energy and focus.

Having cancer teaches you that you are a patient, while most people in the medical industry have no patience for you. Very often you have to sit and wait and do what you are told. Ironically, that becomes one of the keys to healing. If you become anxious over that, you are wasting the little energy you have left to make yourself better.

I relax and laugh a lot more. I enjoy every minute that I am at home, and I don't worry about the endless things that I need to do.

I learned to be "at ease" rather than "in disease."

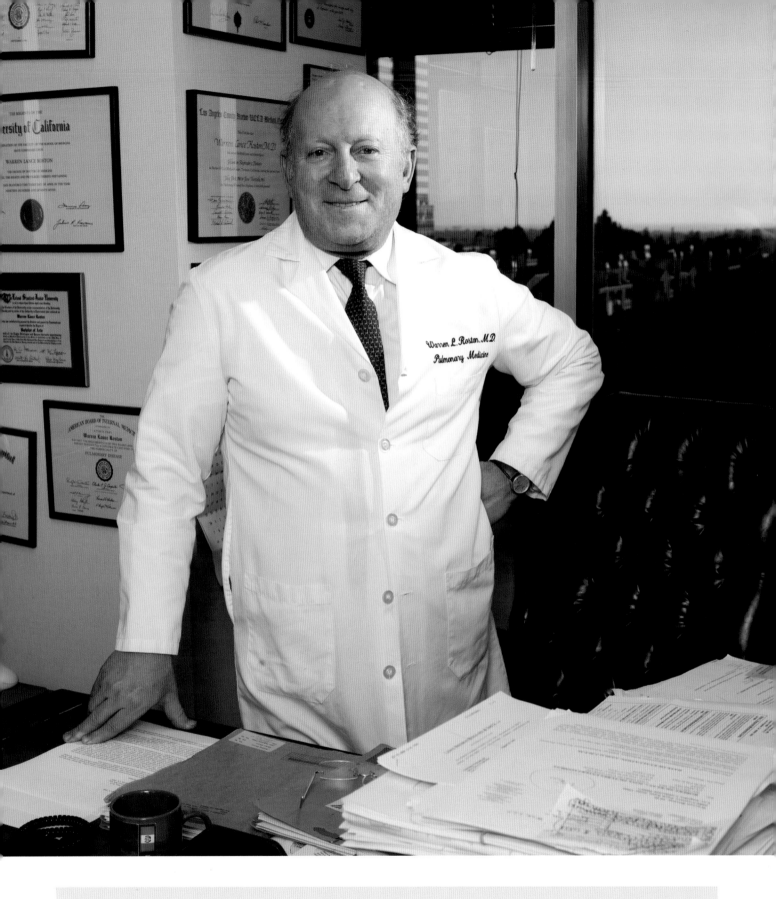

He has always been a great guy. He just went from great to greater.

Warren Roston

Internist, Pulmonary Physician
Age at diagnosis, 55
Metastatic melanoma, 2008

*W*ARREN: The dermatologist I saw told me that he didn't think the bump on my chest was anything to worry about. I told him to take it off right away and biopsy it. It turned out to be melanoma in the subcutaneous tissues, which made it metastatic. Most of my body was heavily involved, including my bones, my kidneys, and my lungs.

I was fortunate because I was able to get to the National Institute of Health. Twenty-four hours later, a physician from the NIH called me and bluntly asked, "Do you want to live? If so, I'll see you in my office in 48 hours."

I thought for about three minutes, called my wife, and the next day we were on a plane. Three days later, I was starting a protocol of interleukin 2 at NIH. It was a long and difficult process of treatments, and each time it felt like a truck hit me . . . no, two trucks.

Being a doctor, I knew what could come, so my fear was increased. I had a pretty deadly disease. Not many survive. They have no way to predict who will do well on interleukin 2, which has about a 5 percent positive response. Half of them recur, so I'm really only one of 3 percent who did well. There must be a God because I can't explain why I'm here. Something dealt me this hand, and then let me win the game.

I learned the importance of human connection and how to receive it. Rather than keeping my illness quiet, I reached out to everyone in the community, hoping they could give me hope and strength. It worked. I tell people now that if they know someone sick, reach out. When in doubt, make the call and just say, "I'm thinking of you." It doesn't matter what you say; just make the call. It was phone calls and emails that got me through the day.

I've become a resource for people newly diagnosed with melanoma. I'm careful what I say, but I know I can help them. That's part of my calling now.

ALISSA, WARREN'S WIFE: As a physician, Warren used to be hesitant to give out-of-office professional advice. Now he is more open and giving of himself. He keeps emphasizing how important it is to give people hope, and I see him doing that on so many levels.

He is an easygoing person. He never sweats the small stuff, and ever since his cancer, I'm now the same way. Small things don't matter. We're here, and that's all that is important. I think his biggest change is that he doesn't work as hard. He comes home earlier and goes out into the garden.

He has always been a great guy. He just went from great to greater.

WARREN: I say to myself, *Hey, I'm here. And it's good to be alive.*

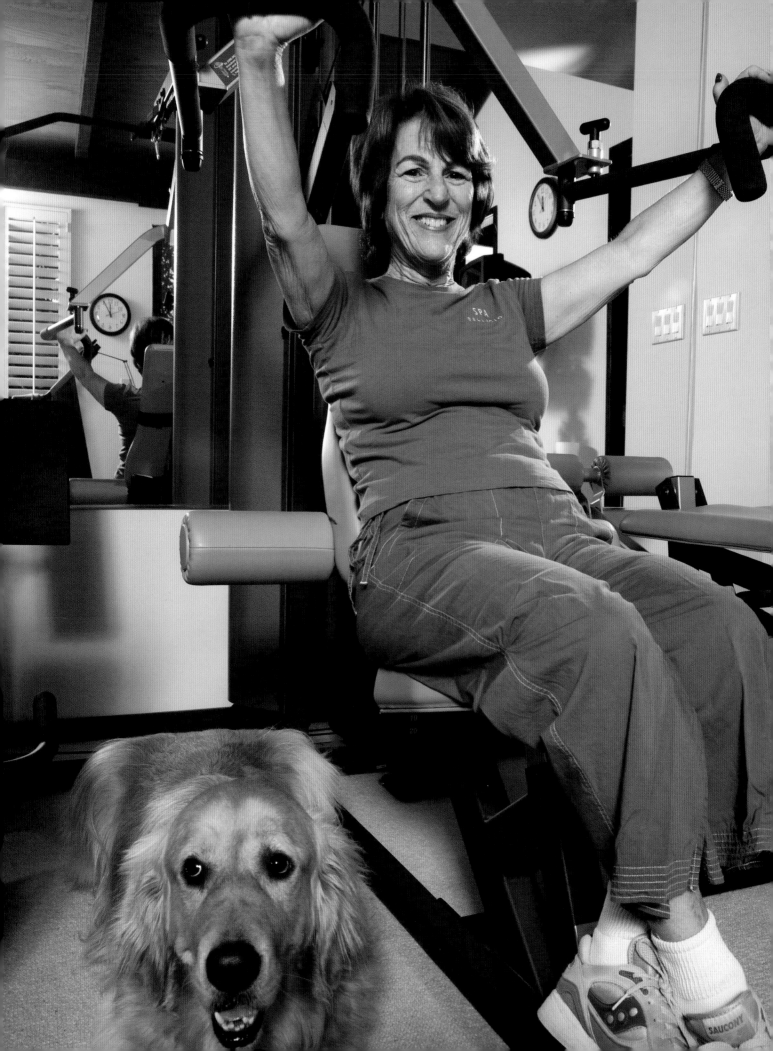

Wendy Ruby
Age at diagnosis, 55
Sarcoma tumor in abdomen, 1997

The doctor told us that, among all the people diagnosed with a sarcoma tumor in the abdomen, 50 percent make it and 50 percent don't. I told my husband I was going to be in the 50 percent that make it. However, there were times during chemo when I wasn't so sure. During one of those chemo treatments, I had a hallucination of my stomach emptying, which I equated with getting rid of my cancer. It was a cleansing feeling. From then on, I knew I was going to make it. One year later, I climbed Machu Picchu with my daughter.

She also introduced me to a healer. He came every week for almost a year, doing Reiki and telling me what he saw. My father died of cancer in 1995, and the healer would see Dad watching over me. He saw the cancer going away and told me it was gone before the CT scans confirmed it. I credit him for making me feel like a person again.

I had a hallucination of my stomach emptying, which I equated with getting rid of my cancer.

Attitude matters. Once you give up, the outcome isn't so terrific. I've always been an optimistic person. Some people carry their cancer with them for a long time, but that's not me. I was never afraid of death. Yes, there were times I thought I might not live, but I wasn't afraid of dying. Whatever happened was okay.

It's hard to believe what I went through. If I hadn't made it, I would have missed seeing my three daughters get married and missed the joy of our adorable granddaughter, as well as all of the other blessings life has offered. Like my father used to say, "If you don't have your health, you don't have anything." I was very lucky to have survived.

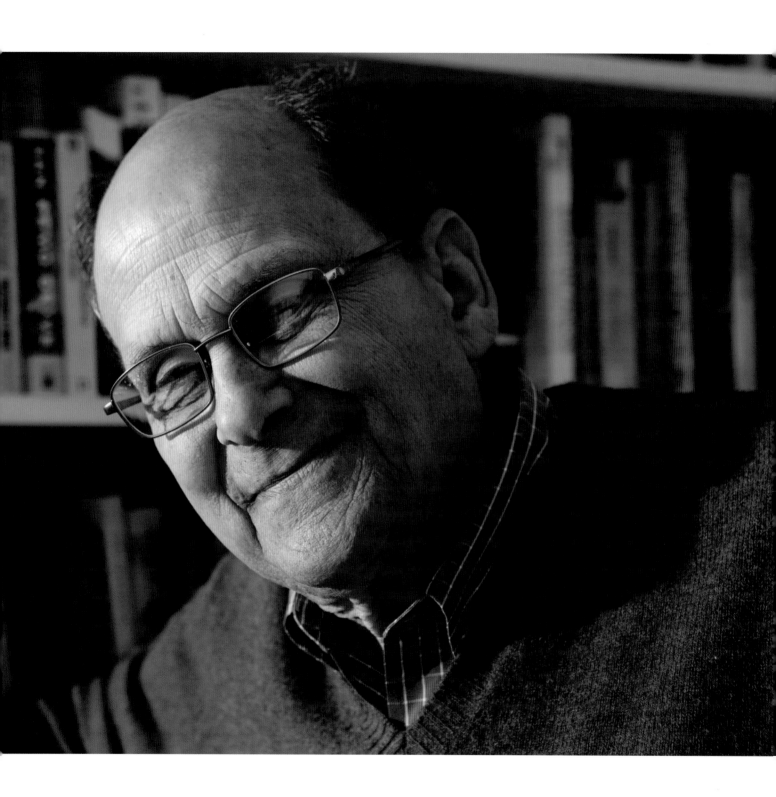

William Cutter

Rabbi, Professor of Hebrew Literature, Hebrew Union College
Age at first heart attack, 41
First heart attack, 1978
Second and third heart attacks, 1992 and 1997
Three angioplasties and two bypass surgeries
Prostate cancer, 2000
Recurrence, 2007

I've been through four life-threatening situations; a couple of those were very dramatic. But oddly enough, I don't feel fragile in the day to day of living. Other things have become more important than my illnesses, especially my relationships with others and my work.

I do admit that my health history increased my sensitivity to the fact of illness in our world and to the need to assist others as they go through their inevitable health crises. That is one of the reasons I began working with my rabbinic students on pastoral service through UCLA Medical Center and Cedars Sinai Hospital in Los Angeles. Eventually my school helped establish the Kalsman Institute on Judaism and Health—a project devoted to serving the frail and ill, and a consciousness-raiser for Jewish institutions throughout the United States and Israel.

My emotional reaction to all of this is a special joy that I am alive. Objectively, I see that life is always precarious, but that we needn't feel that living is dangerous. I especially accept that my life will be shortened from some imagined and ideal age, but actually I am free of any worries about that. I continue to want to serve some good purpose in this area of human experience.

> *I continue to want to serve some good purpose in this area of human experience.*

Rabbi William Cutter, PhD, is Steinberg Emeritus Professor of Human Relations at Hebrew Union College – Jewish Institute of Religion, where he held the Paul and Trudy Steinberg Chair in Human Relations and was Professor of Modern Hebrew Literature and Education. He was Founding Director of HUC—JIR's Rhea Hirsch School of Education and the Kalsman Institute on Judaism and Health.

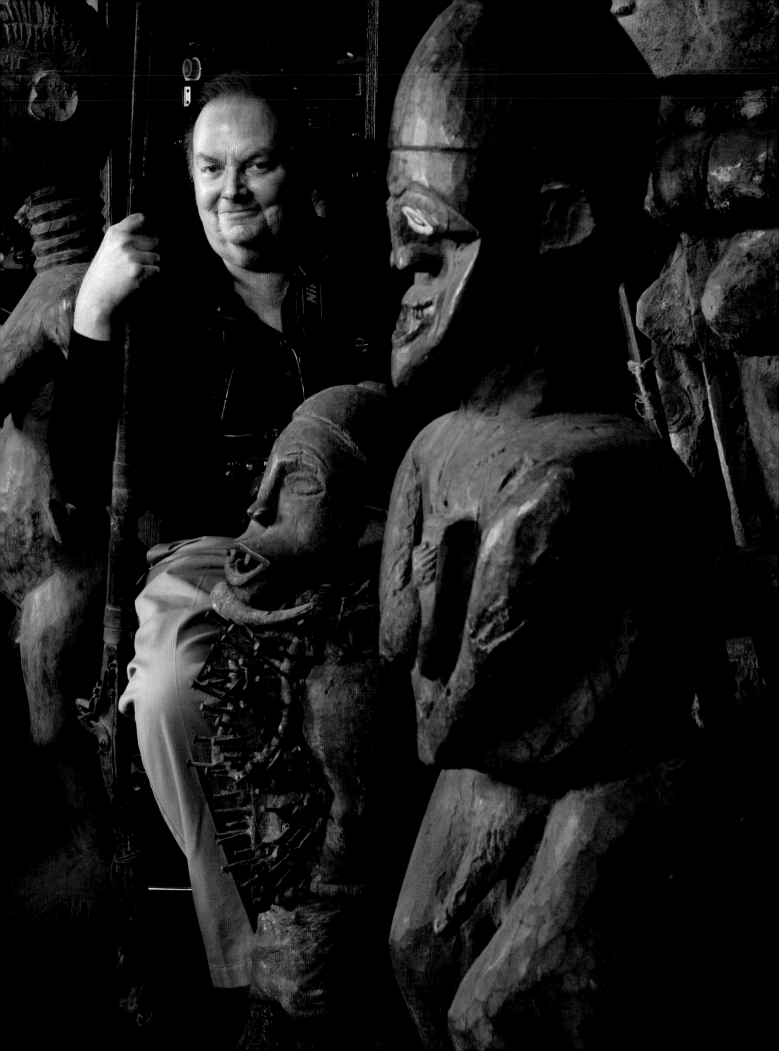

William Ericson

Photographer, Publisher of *South Pasadena Review* and *Quarterly Magazine*
Age at diagnosis, 63
Multiple myeloma, 2007

riginally, when the doctors gave me twenty-five days to live, I thought, *What can I accomplish in twenty-five days?* I called for an appointment with an oncologist and was told he couldn't see me for a month. I told him that would be too late.

Treatment was difficult for me. Chemotherapy was working until a lidocaine shot, given simply to lance a cyst, caused Stevens-Johnson syndrome. I spent six weeks in the hospital and lost my skin completely down to the flesh.

Of course I immediately started thinking about my legacy. I've always been a fighter. So I decided I wanted to fight for all the people who have been good to me. I started a foundation to keep everyone employed at my magazine and newspaper after I am gone. I also started producing a book of my photography, which is another part of my legacy. Since I don't have children, this book is my child. I have since sold the newspaper and magazine, but still remain editorial consultant and photographer.

> . . . I decided I wanted to fight for all the people who have been good to me.

I've had many jobs. I began photographing in junior high school when I learned that if you point a camera at beautiful women, you get their attention. I eventually ended up shooting celebrities for all the major studios. In 1978 I took over the family newspaper. I was also a music rep for many years for lots of big bands. I am also a collector of African art.

I've had several lives in this life, and when this one is over, I'll have had more fun than most people.

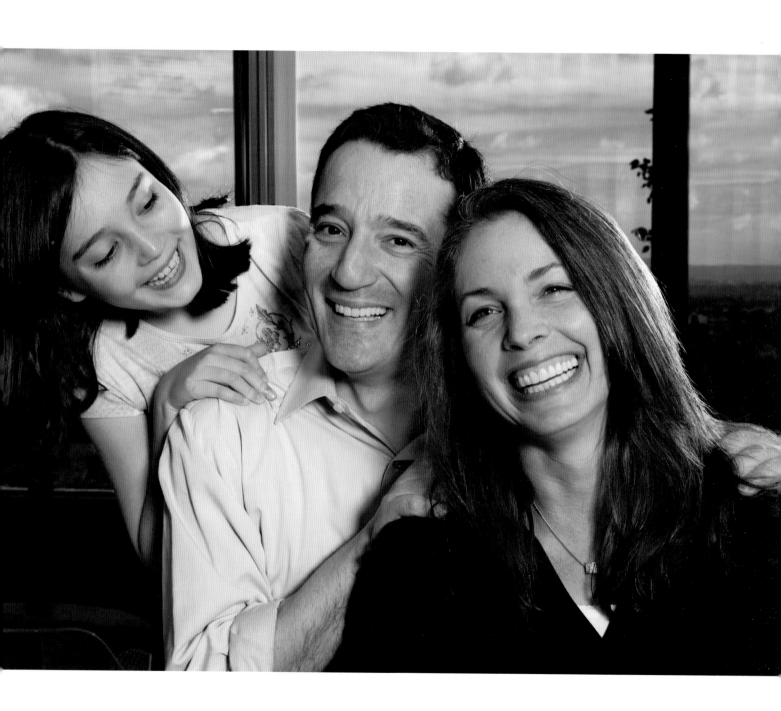

David Wolpe

Congregational Rabbi, Author of Seven Books
Age at first diagnosis, 44
Grand mal seizure, benign brain tumor, 2003
Follicular non-Hodgkin's lymphoma, 2006

EILEEN handled her cancer by researching and finding out as much as she could. I handled it by letting the doctors take care of it.

As a rabbi, I have the privilege of being surrounded by significant moments in people's lives. I handled cancer the way I handle almost every experience. I turned it into a teaching. I process events by finding ways to speak about them. As I was going into chemo, I prayed, "Let me get a sermon out of this." After all, if I can't get a sermon out of having cancer, I'm a poor excuse for a rabbi. Every time I walk into a hospital room, my cancer is an odd blessing, because the patients know I have been there. I understand.

Cancer confirmed that I was leading the life I should be living. It settled me into my job and my life, allowing me to treasure them like never before.

The playwright Eugène Ionesco said, "Everything in life is expressible in words except the living truth." What you learn from an experience like this is inexpressible. It's the deepest message and meaning of life.

What you learn from an experience like this is inexpressible. It's the deepest message and meaning of life.

Here is a story that could only happen in Los Angeles. While I was bald, a guy come up to me and said, "I know how you feel because in two movies I was a stunt double for Patrick Stewart."

Eileen Ansel Wolpe

Editor, Silversmith, Mother
Age at diagnosis, 31
Endocervical adenocarcinoma in situ, 1997

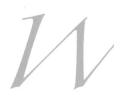

We had just moved to Los Angeles with a six-month-old daughter, and I knew something wasn't right. Looking back, I feel like there was an angel who whispered, "Go to the doctor." I had eight "skip" lesions and a rare, aggressive form of reproductive carcinoma, in situ. If I had waited two weeks longer to heed the warning, I might not be sitting here right now.

The day after my thirty-second birthday, I had a modified radical hysterectomy. When I left the hospital, they told me to lead my normal life as if nothing had changed. For me that was not an option. I knew something needed to change. I felt a desperate need to gain some kind of control. What I learned is that the only control I can really have in my life is how I choose to respond to the things that happen to me. Instead of an automatic reaction, if I can take a moment, stay centered, and "be in me," my quality of life skyrockets. I learned to respond instead of just reacting.

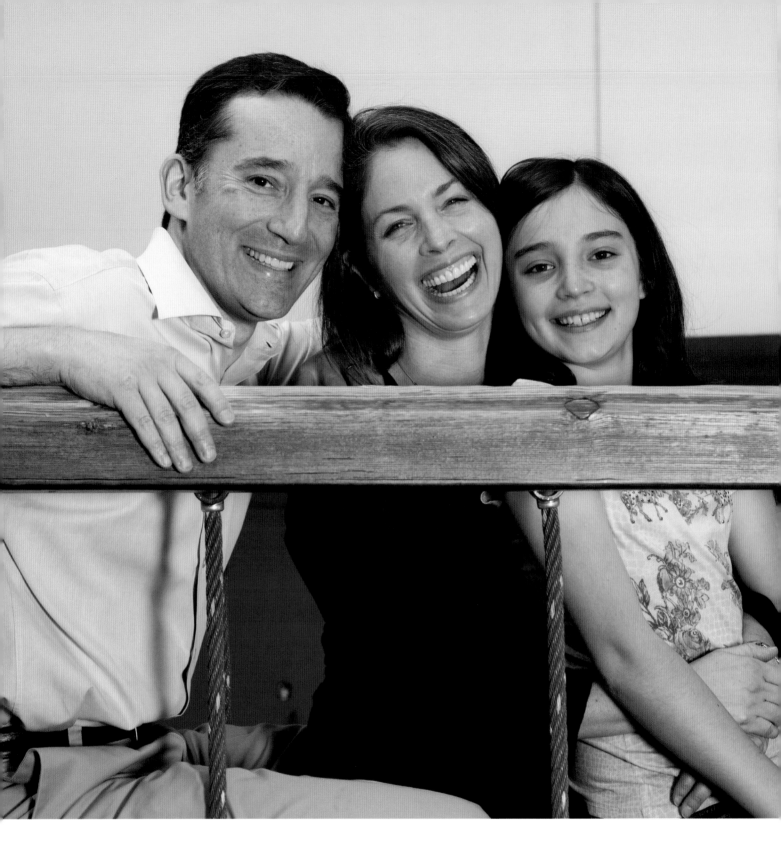

When it was clear that our daughter was going to be our only child, there was no way I was giving up a moment of time with her. But for me, the most precious part of every day was to be with my baby when she went to sleep at night. I didn't miss a single night those first ten years. Not one.

Cancer is a thief, and the first thing it steals is your youth. Your naiveté. Your fantasy of immortality. In its place it leaves a gift: the knowledge of limited time, of mortality, and the clarity of what matters.

Six years after my diagnosis, David was diagnosed with a brain tumor that presented with a grand mal seizure. And three years after that, he was diagnosed with follicular non-Hodgkin's lymphoma. David and I have now played both sides, cancer patient and caretaker. It's beyond terrifying to be the patient, but it is far more anxiety making to be the caretaker.

In many ways, cancer is a "get out of jail free" card. It taught me to prioritize my life. It taught me what matters most. And what matters least. For the first time in my life I felt free to say no to individuals and to things that were not healthy for me.

It leaves a gift: the knowledge of limited time, of mortality, and the clarity of what matters.

I survived. I am one of the lucky ones.

SAMARA WOLPE, 13 YEARS OLD: I'll never forget the feeling of waking up and knowing that your parent has cancer. Sometimes I look at all the other kids and think they are lucky because they don't have to go through this. But I also feel like it's made me stronger, and they don't understand that. When I look at people now, I wonder about their lives. I wonder if they understand.

Once you have suffered, you look for other people who can understand that feeling. Having a parent with cancer separates you from the other kids your age. When I am at school or in some other setting where there are kids, I look for people who are able to relate to the kinds of things I have experienced. It helps to have that common ground in a friend.

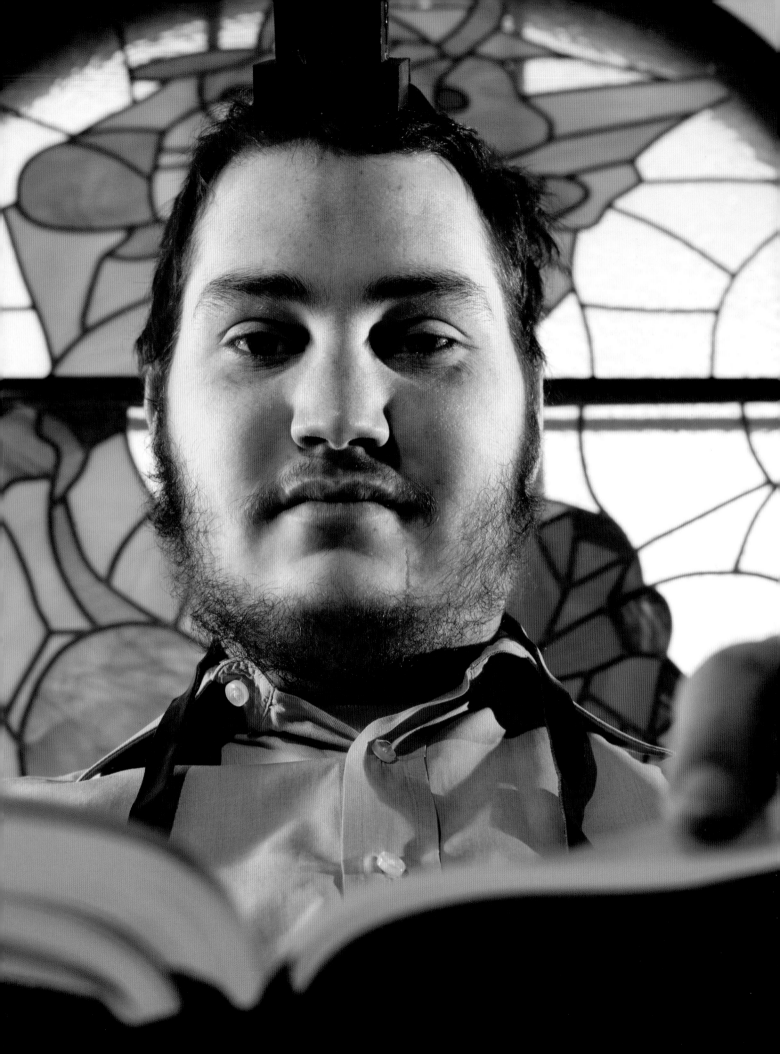

Yosef Eliezrie

Rabbi; Web Development, Chabad.org
Age at diagnosis, 19
Acute myelogenous leukemia, 2005

I was nineteen years old and planning my life. I was one of 100 students selected to go to Lithuania for a summer outreach program. While there, I got very sick. My white blood count was 100 times normal. The flight home was very difficult, but that is where I met my first angel. A woman from Hawaii sitting in the next seat took care of me.

The next thing I remember was waking up in the ICU. I had been unconscious for nine days. The doctor told my father I was not going to make it. I was the first adult that they had ever treated with nitrous oxide, a drug used for premature babies. It saved my life. During that time, I had a dream that I was on a boat between two islands, life and death.

In March they told me I was in remission, but then in August the cancer was back. It was worse this time. I needed a bone marrow transplant; they found a one-in-a-million donor match, a twenty-four-year-old man in Jerusalem. He was my second angel. He proved that there are amazingly selfless people in this world. What do you say to someone like that?

Leukemia is the worst and best thing that ever happened to me. I have learned so much. I thought my whole life, my whole world, was planned and I knew who all my friends were. Then I met these angels. The world is filled with amazing people. I took what others gave me, especially their positive outlook, and am trying to apply that to my own life. There is still a lot of good to be done in the world, and I want to do my part.

I wear this wristband every single day. It is a red band from the Leukemia and Lymphoma Society representing a drop of blood. My night nurse gave it to me and said, "I wish for you to live by this." And I do. I was nineteen years old then. God decided to make me better, and He did it for a reason. My life is a whole different story. I don't waste time. I make the most of every day. Every morning I say, "What can I do for the world today because God has given me the gift of life again."

> *"What can I do for the world today because God has given me the gift of life again."*

INDEX

CANCERS SORTED BY GROUP

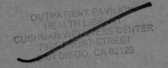